Dance Medicine

Editor

KATHLEEN L. DAVENPORT

PHYSICAL MEDICINE AND REHABILITATION CLINICS OF NORTH AMERICA

www.pmr.theclinics.com

Consulting Editor
SANTOS F. MARTINEZ

February 2021 • Volume 32 • Number 1

ELSEVIER

1600 John F. Kennedy Boulevard • Suite 1800 • Philadelphia, Pennsylvania, 19103-2899

http://www.theclinics.com

PHYSICAL MEDICINE AND REHABILITATION CLINICS OF NORTH AMERICA Volume 32, Number 1
February 2021 ISSN 1047-9651, 978-0-323-75992-2

Editor: Lauren Boyle
Developmental Editor: Nicole Congleton

Reprints. For copies of 100 or more of articles in this publication, please contact the Commercial Reprints Department, Elsevier Inc., 360 Park Avenue South, New York, NY 10010-1710. Tel.: 212-633-3874; Fax: 212-633-3820; E-mail: reprints@elsevier.com.

Physical Medicine and Rehabilitation Clinics of North America (ISSN 1047-9651) is published quarterly by Elsevier Inc., 360 Park Avenue South, New York, NY 10010-1710. Months of issue are February, May, August, and November. Business and Editorial Offices: 1600 John F. Kennedy Blvd., Suite 1800, Philadelphia, PA 19103-2899. Customer Service Office: 3251 Riverport Lane, Maryland Heights, MO 63043. Periodicals postage paid at New York, NY and additional mailing offices. Subscription price per year is $322.00 (US individuals), $879.00 (US institutions), $100.00 (US students), $366.00 (Canadian individuals), $923.00 (Canadian institutions), $100.00 (Canadian students), $463.00 (foreign individuals), $923.00 (foreign institutions), and $210.00 (foreign students). Foreign air speed delivery is included in all *Clinics* subscription prices. All prices are subject to change without notice. **POSTMASTER:** Send address changes to *Physical Medicine and Rehabilitation Clinics of North America*, Customer Service Office: Elsevier Health Sciences Division, Subscription Customer Service, 3251 Riverport Lane, Maryland Heights, MO 63043. **Customer Service: 1-800-654-2452 (US). From outside of the United States, call 314-447-8871. Fax: 314-447-8029. E-mail: JournalsCustomer Service-usa@elsevier.com (for print support); JournalsOnlineSupport-usa@elsevier.com (for online support).**

Physical Medicine and Rehabilitation Clinics of North America is indexed in *Excerpta Medica, MEDLINE/PubMed (Index Medicus), Cinahl,* and *Cumulative Index to Nursing and Allied Health Literature.*

Contributors

CONSULTING EDITOR

SANTOS F. MARTINEZ, MD, MS
Dance Medicine: Ballet Memphis, Physical Medicine and Rehabilitation, Campbell Clinic, Assistant Professor, Department of Orthopaedics, University of Tennessee School of Medicine, Memphis, Tennessee, USA

EDITOR

KATHLEEN L. DAVENPORT, MD
Director of Physiatry, Hospital for Special Surgery Florida, West Palm Beach, Florida, USA

AUTHORS

JATIN P. AMBEGAONKAR, PhD, ATC, OT, CSCS, FIADMS
Sports Medicine Assessment Research and Testing (SMART) Laboratory, George Mason University, Manassas, Virginia, USA

BENÉ BARRERA, BS, ATC
Athletic Training Coordinator, Houston Methodist Orthopedics and Sports Medicine, Houston, Texas, USA

DAN BENARDOT, PhD, DHC, RD, LD, FACSM
Professor of Practice, Center for the Study of Human Health, Candler Library, Emory University, Professor of Nutrition, Emeritus, Georgia State University, Atlanta, Georgia, USA

AMANDA M. BLACKMON, PT, DPT
Board Certified Orthopeadic Clinical Specialist, Certified Myofascial Trigger Point Therapist, Adjunct Clinical Assistant Professor, Department of Physical Therapy, College of Health Professions, Mercer University, Instructor, Myopain Seminars, Head Physical Therapist, Atlanta Ballet, Partner, Atlanta Dance Medicine, CEO, MandyDancePT, LLC, Atlanta, Georgia, USA

KATHLEEN BOWER, PT, DPT
Director of Dance Medicine, Miami City Ballet, Miami Beach, Florida, USA

ANN F. BROWN, PhD, CISSN
Human Performance Laboratory, Department of Movement Sciences, University of Idaho, College of Education Health and Human Sciences, Moscow, Idaho, USA

LILLIAN CHONG, BS, ACSM-EP
Sports Medicine Assessment Research and Testing (SMART) Laboratory, George Mason University, Manassas, Virginia, USA

MARY DUBON, MD
Instructor in Physical Medicine and Rehabilitation, Pediatric Rehabilitation Medicine Attending Physician and Pediatric Sports Medicine Attending Physician, Boston Children's Hospital, Spaulding Rehabilitation Hospital, Harvard Medical School, Boston, Massachusetts, USA

LAUREN ELSON, MD
Director of Dance Medicine, Spaulding Rehabilitation, Physical Medicine and Rehabilitation, Instructor, Harvard Medical School, Boston, Massachusetts, USA

EMMA FAULKNER, PT, DPT, OCS
Atlanta Dance Medicine, TriHealth Physical Therapy, LLC, Atlanta Ballet, Department of Theater and Dance, Emory University, Decatur, Georgia, USA

ALEX Y. HAN, MD
Medical Resident, Houston Methodist Orthopedics and Sports Medicine, Houston, Texas, USA

MELODY HRUBES, MD
Director, Non-Operative Sports Medicine, Rothman Orthopaedics, Medical Director, Radio City Rockettes, New York, New York, USA

JENNIFER JANOWSKI, PT, DScPT, OCS, FAAOMPT
Athletico Physical Therapy, Physical Therapist, Joffrey Ballet, Chicago, Illinois, USA

PRANJAL JOSHI, MS
Sports Medicine Assessment Research and Testing (SMART) Laboratory, George Mason University, Manassas, Virginia, USA

CAROLYN E. KEELER, DO
Department of Neurosurgery, Assistant Professor, Duke University Medical Center, Durham, North Carolina, USA

LAUREN McINTYRE, ATC
Clinical Specialist and Athletic Trainer, Harkness Center for Dance Injuries at NYU Langone Health, New York, New York, USA

MERRY LYNN MORRIS, MFA, PhD
Assistant Director, Dance Program, School of Theatre and Dance College of the Arts, University of South Florida, Tampa, Florida, USA

CARINA M. NASRALLAH, MS, ATC
Outreach Athletic Trainer, Houston Methodist Orthopedics and Sports Medicine, Houston, Texas, USA

DAVID M. POPOLI, MD
Assistant Professor, Departments of Orthopedics and Pediatrics, Divisions of PM&R and Sports Medicine, Wake Forest Baptist Health, Winston Salem, North Carolina, USA

BRIDGET J. QUINN, MD
Division of Sports Medicine, Department of Orthopedic Surgery, Boston Children's Hospital, Boston, Massachusetts, USA

JEFFREY A. RUSSELL, PhD, AT, FIADMS
Associate Professor of Athletic Training and Director of Science and Health in Artistic Performance, Ohio University, College of Health Sciences and Professions, School of Applied Health Sciences and Wellness, Athens, Ohio, USA

CHARLES SCOTT, MD
Division of Sports Medicine, Department of Orthopedic Surgery, Boston Children's Hospital, Boston, Massachusetts, USA

SELINA SHAH, MD, FACP, FAMSSM
A Division of BASS Medical Group, Walnut Creek, California, USA; Dance Company Physician for Diablo Ballet, Contra Costa Ballet, New Ballet, San Jose, California, USA; Team Physician for USA Artistic Swimming, Colorado Springs, Colorado, USA

REBECCA SIEGEL, MD
Pediatric Rehabilitation Medicine Fellow, Spaulding Rehabilitation Hospital, Harvard Medical School, Boston, Massachusetts, USA

JUDITH SMITH
Founding Member and Artistic Director Emerita, AXIS Dance Company, Oakland, California, USA

LORI STEWART, BPE
Health and Safety Performer Advocate, Union of British Columbia Performers/ACTRA, Vancouver, British Columbia, Canada

ANDREA STRACCIOLINI, MD, FAAP, FACSM
Division of Sports Medicine, Department of Orthopedic Surgery, Boston Children's Hospital, Boston, Massachusetts, USA

MARK TOMASIC, MFA
Associate Professor of Dance, Santa Monica College, Artistic Advisor, Dancing Wheels Company & School, California, USA

KEVIN E. VARNER, MD
Director of Orthopedics, Houston Methodist Orthopedics and Sports Medicine, Houston, Texas, USA

TINA WANG, MD
Associate Professor, Loma Linda School of Medicine, Attending Physician, Loma Linda VA Hospital, Upland, California, USA

Contents

> Rehabilitation of dance injury should be a team-based approach lead by a medical practitioner with experience in both musculoskeletal medicine and dance specific demands. The rehabilitation protocol begins with a dance specific initial assessment, followed by injury management, progression of the rehabilitation program including dance specific movement, advancing to full independence.

> Dancers require a unique blend of artistry and athleticism, and have specific medical problems that require the expertise of health care professionals who understand the demands of the performing arts. There is often a lack of alignment between health care systems and dancers' perceptions of care. Factors including country of residence, socioeconomic status, and local infrastructure can affect dancers' access to health care. Efforts to improve access are evident, and specialized care for dancers has grown significantly in recent decades. By developing and refining systems of care delivery, there are opportunities to ensure optimal health of the dancer population.

> Dancers represent a unique subset of athletes who face physical and psychological stressors throughout their careers. These challenges pose risks for injury, burnout, and diminished performance capacity. This article proposes a proactive intervention. The Active Resilience Training in Dance curriculum would provide dancers with useable instruction at key career inflection points (amateur to preprofessional, preprofessional to professional, and professional to retirement) to bolster the 4 pillars of their resilience (emotional, cognitive, spiritual, and physical).

> Performing artists are similar to sports athletes, with repeated patterns of training and performing. This requires that artistic athletes manage the

dynamic interaction between energy/nutrient/fluid utilization and provision to assure long, healthful, and successful careers. Although sports athletes have an abundance of science-based nutritional guidance available, there are few nutrition-focused resources available to artistic athletes, which can result in failure to optimally satisfy the artistic athlete's individual nutritional needs. The purpose of this article is to review common nutritional issues faced by artistic athletes and to present science-based nutrition strategies that can aid in lowering nutrition-associated health and performance risks.

Dancers' energy demands fluctuate across the season. Accordingly, dancers should adapt their training and nutrition. Still, how to periodize nutrition in dancers remains unclear. This article aims to (1) introduce nutrition periodization and (2) provide recommendations for nutrition periodization in dancers. During preseason, dancers design, rehearse, and train. During in-season, dancers have one or more daily performances. During postseason, dancers rest and prepare for the next season. Nutrition periodization is the strategic and timed nutrient intake to meet varying seasonal energy demands. Overall, nutrition periodization can support dancers' training goals, enhance their performance, and support optimal recovery.

Care of young dancers requires a unique approach during a critical time of growth and development. Young dancers' well-being depends on factors including sleep, mental health, growth-associated musculoskeletal imbalances, and nutrition. Puberty is a particularly important time for young dancers. It coincides with an increased commitment to their art form and physical/psychosocial changes. It is imperative for practitioners to understand these various factors in order to optimize young dancers' health and allow them to safely train and perform.

Advancing to pointe requires sufficient maturity, strength, and flexibility and adequate ballet training to develop the skills which usually occurs between the ages 11 and 13. Health practitioners can provide studios with an objective assessment to determine if a young dancer is ready to transition to en pointe. The evaluator should be proficient in ballet, because the evaluation largely is dance based and includes a history and physical examination as well as a comprehensive assessment. The plan includes health improvement tips and summarizes technique flaws as well as exercises to improve these and other deficits. The goal is to transition dancers safely to pointe.

Because of increased choreographic demands, early specialization, multi-genre dancers, and high incidence of career-ending injuries, there is a need for enhanced training methodologies to address the unique needs of today's professional dancer. It is imperative for company directors, instructors, choreographers, and dance medicine practitioners to consider implementing the most specific conditioning and training programs to prepare their dancers to meet or exceed expectations without resultant injury. Quantifying effectiveness of choreography-specific training programs is an area for further research. The implementation of scientific principles can and should be used to enhance dancers' health, performance, athleticism, and artistry.

Dancing, like athletics, is physically demanding, but dancing also involves aesthetics. Although athletes often use supplemental training, little information exists about its use in dancers. A review of types and effects of supplemental training on dancers' performance and injury risk indicates that, among largely female collegiate dancers, supplemental training enhances the dancers' performance, but limited evidence exists for injury risk reduction.

Thirty years ago the introduction of on-site health care for professional dance companies was a novel concept and dance medicine clinicians often had limited on-site hours, restricted treatment space, and small budgets. Companies are now developing fully staffed on-site clinics and backstage care that provide a multidisciplinary approach to dancer health and wellness. On-site dance medicine programs focus on holistic dancer health and preventive care rather than just triage and rehabilitation. Best practice recommendations for care of professional dancer patients allow for streamlined patient care within a network of medical professionals who understand the demands of a professional dance career.

Dancers and other performing artists are subject to head impacts that result in concussion-like symptoms. In spite of this, performing arts do not have access to the continual, focused emphasis on the diagnosis, management, and prevention of concussions that is commonplace in sports. Performing arts present a unique environment in which concussions occur and must be managed. This article outlines what is known about performing arts concussions, describes mechanisms of head impacts sustained by participants in dance and the related artforms of theater, circus, and film and television stunts, and offers concussion management guidelines for these artistic fields.

Dancers frequently present to health care professionals with musculoskeletal impairments. The role of the health care practitioner, whether physician, physical therapist, or acupuncturist, is to decrease pain and restore function in the short term and to restore adaptive potential and neural connectivity in the long term. When dysfunction is treated, pain improves. Acupuncture and dry needling improve tissue perfusion by improving vasomotor control and can improve strength by removing motor inhibition. Acupuncture and dry needling are safe, complementary modalities aimed at improving the function of the dancer.

This article explores relevant issues in dance medicine for dancers with disabilities, blindness/low vision, and/or deafness/hard of hearing (DWDBD). Within dance medicine and science, there has been minimal focus on DWDBD. Little is known about injury patterns, injury prevention, or wellness strategies for DWDBD. However, there are increasing numbers of dance programs and companies involving DWDBD at preprofessional and professional levels. This article reviews the history and experience of DWDBD and offers best guidance regarding dance medicine considerations for DWDBD based on the limited research and evidence that exists, extrapolation from para/adaptive sports medicine literature, and expert opinion.

PHYSICAL MEDICINE AND REHABILITATION CLINICS OF NORTH AMERICA

SERIES OF RELATED INTEREST

Orthopedic Clinics
Clinics in Sports Medicine
Neurologic Clinics

VISIT THE CLINICS ONLINE!
Access your subscription at:
www.theclinics.com

Foreword
Dance is Art

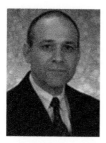

Santos F. Martinez, MD, MS
Consulting Editor

I appreciate Dr Davenport's willingness to take on this project for a unique field of athletes whose lives are dedicated to the Arts. Their commitment to this craft is exemplified by an initiation and training typically in early childhood. There are developmental adaptations of one's body and mind to such rigorous cycles of conditioning as the dancer progresses from childhood to adolescence and possibly to the elite professional ranks. Attributes from dancing become part of one's spirit and life whether they train at the amateur or professional levels.

Care for these athletes requires a multitude of resources from physician and allied health specialists extending to psychologists, nutritionists, body workers with a knowledge of biomechanics, exercise physiology, and the consequences of injuries. Dr Davenport's approach is certainly a welcome asset to the field as it serves as an adjunct to other resources in Dance Medicine. We are indebted to the medical professionals, instructors, volunteers, and contributors who dedicate countless hours to this patient population. I also wish to personally thank Dr Greer Richardson for his 33 years of service to the dance community at Campbell Clinic in Memphis, Tennessee.

Santos F. Martinez, MD, MS
Dance Medicine: Ballet Memphis
Physical Medicine and Rehabilitation
Campbell Clinic
Department of Orthopaedics
University of Tennessee School of Medicine
Memphis, TN 38104, USA

E-mail address:
smartinez@campbellclinic.com

Phys Med Rehabil Clin N Am 32 (2021) xiii
https://doi.org/10.1016/j.pmr.2020.09.012
1047-9651/21/© 2020 Published by Elsevier Inc.

Preface

Dance Medicine for the Physiatrist

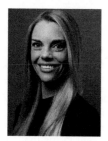

Kathleen L. Davenport, MD
Editor

Performing arts and dance medicine is an important topic for physiatrists. Many dancers and performing artists look to our specialty for diagnosis and management with their hope to avoid surgery. They may enter our clinics in fear of a career-ending injury or a provider who does not understand their unique medical needs. It is hoped that this issue will supplement clinical tools and pearls to optimize treatment of our artistic athletes.

Many concepts of performing arts and dance medicine are found in traditional athletics. The information presented allows clinical application to this unique population. Many dancers report feeling uncertain that their physician understands their unique needs and requirements of their sport. Physiatrists are well positioned to diagnose and manage these artistic athletes through their training, focused on individualized care and movement specific rehabilitation. For example, concussion management of traditional athletes can be tailored to address the issues of stage lighting and rotational movement patterns, such as frequent turns. In addition, functional movement-specific adaptations can be honed for our disabled dancers.

Unfortunately, there is a paucity of research in dancers and performing artists when compared with traditional athletes. Therefore, much of the literature presented in this supplement combines athletic literature with the smaller volume of dance and performing arts research and clinical knowledge. At times, the work presented in the following articles is the first time this information has been published in the literature. While these issues have been widely discussed within our small dance and performing arts communities, at times this information has not extended into the wider accessibility of publication. It is hoped that these topics will advance scientific conversations and research directions to continue to build the body of dance and performing arts literature.

This supplement in dance and performing arts medicine highlights clinical topics as a tool in the treatment of the artistic athlete. There are other excellent resources that have taken a "body part" approach to the dancer, and the intent of the current

Phys Med Rehabil Clin N Am 32 (2021) xv–xvi
https://doi.org/10.1016/j.pmr.2020.09.011
1047-9651/21/© 2020 Published by Elsevier Inc.

publication is to complement with a functional approach. The importance of mental health and nutrition cannot be overstated in this population, as with our traditional athletes. These themes are highlighted and pervasive throughout this supplement. In addition, the authors outline many clinical tools to consider in the diagnosis of performing artists, including screening tools for dancers. In the clinical management of artistic athletes, the authors discuss options, such as needling and biomechanical feedback, for this unique population, who at times seeks "alternative" approaches to their health care. This supplement offers its readers options to best serve our performing artists and dancers.

I want to personally thank the contributing authors for their bravery and work to come together for this "performance." Brava!

Kathleen L. Davenport, MD
Hospital for Special Surgery Florida
300 Palm Beach Lakes Boulevard
West Palm Beach, FL 33401, USA

E-mail address:
davenportk@hss.edu

Rehabilitation of the Dancer

Melody Hrubes, MD[a],*, Jennifer Janowski, PT, DScPT, OCS, FAAOMPT[b]

KEYWORDS

- Dance progression • Dance recovery • Dance injury management
- Dance rehabilitation

KEY POINTS

- Rehabilitation of a dance injury should be a team-based approach led by a medical practitioner with experience in both musculoskeletal medicine and the specific demands placed on a dancer's body and psyche.
- Rehabilitation protocol begins with assessment and diagnosis of injury, followed by injury management.
- Progression of the rehabilitation program for a dancer includes dance specific movement, such as turn-out, balance progression, turn progression, jump progression, and partnering and lifting.
- The goal of a dance-specific rehabilitation protocol is to successfully return the dancer to their previous level of function.

INTRODUCTION

The annual incidence of injury in professional dancers ranges from 67% to 95%.[1] The goal of dance rehabilitation is to address the cause of injury and prepare the dancer for a successful return to previous level of function while minimizing reinjury. Often, an injured dancer can fully recover with improved skills and a decreased injury risk. Dance-specific rehabilitation is of paramount importance to achieving the best possible outcome.[2]

Rehabilitation of a dance injury should be a team-based approach led by a medical practitioner with experience in both musculoskeletal medicine and the specific demands placed on a dancer's body and psyche. Dance requires a sport-specific vocabulary that should be used to ensure optimal communication. Depending on the injury type, the rehabilitation team may include physicians, physical or occupational therapists, athletic trainers, massage therapists, nutritionists and/or dieticians, psychiatrists and/or psychologists, chiropractors, podiatrists, acupuncturists, and other somatic practitioners. Dance teachers or artistic directors may also be involved. When available, the in-house medical team provides valuable insight into the demands of the company and the dancer's premorbid function and is involved in the transition

[a] Rothman Orthopaedics, 645 Madison Avenue, New York, NY 10022, USA; [b] Athletico Physical Therapy, 24 E. Chicago Ave, Chicago, IL 60611, USA
* Corresponding
E-mail address: melodyhrubes@gmail.com

Phys Med Rehabil Clin N Am 32 (2021) 1–20
https://doi.org/10.1016/j.pmr.2020.08.003
1047-9651/21/© 2020 Elsevier Inc. All rights reserved.

of care to full dance activity. A dancer might not have access to an onsite medical team, so dance staff and physician may communicate directly regarding appropriate activity level. The composition of the rehabilitation team adapts to best address the injury and contributing factors.

The rehabilitation process must address both intrinsic and extrinsic contributions to the injury to maximize the potential for successful return to dance. Intrinsic risk factors for injury, such as age and growth, strength imbalance, inadequate flexibility, malalignment, or incorrect biomechanics and technique, can often lead to overuse injuries or contribute to traumatic dance injuries.[3] Dancers more commonly suffer from overuse injuries (65%), but traumatic injuries are a significant concern (35%).[4] Extrinsic risk factors for injury include the dancer's environment and can lead to traumatic injuries, such as a poorly lit staircase causing a dancer to fall down the stairs, loose costuming causing a dropped lift, or slippery shoe soles causing a fall. These extrinsic factors are important to identify, as they remain a recurrent injury risk for that dancer and a new injury risk to other dancers. Other extrinsic factors include dance style, props, stage type and flooring, and amount of training per season.[3]

DANCE MEDICINE REHABILITATION PROGRESSION PROTOCOL

Dance injuries require a multifactorial approach to management. This rehabilitation progression protocol for dance medicine (**Table 1**)[5] integrates multiple aspects to address. Because every injury is unique, different stages may blend, as some aspects progress faster than others. This table provides a generalized tool that can be tailored to each individual rehabilitation plan. Throughout the rehabilitation process, it is critical to keep the dancer dancing and integrated into the company or class as allowed by limitations of the injury. In dance, as other sports, ceasing all activity for a period of time without addressing underlying causes of injury is seldom successful and can create distrust between athlete and medical profession.

Set Expectations

Share a typical timeframe for return to dance after a specific injury, understanding that each injury is unique. Be honest regarding the estimated time to return to dance. This allows the dancer and company to plan for short-term and long-term future. In addition, clarify the dancer's previous level of dancing, upcoming performances or auditions, future expectation, and functional goals. A dancer who plans to be a professional has different requirements than the dancer who wishes to attend class recreationally. This step is necessary early in the rehabilitation process, as inaccurate expectations are associated with decreased satisfaction and increased pain after injury.[6]

Proper participation in their rehabilitation process is multifactorial and expectations should be discussed. This may include being well rested and mentally prepared for therapy sessions, ensuring proper and adequate nutrition for healing, and complying with home exercises. The dancer needs to be aware that progression will occur as specific targets are met. In some aspects, foundational work must be done, which can be perceived as basic and boring.

Communication throughout the rehabilitation process between the dancer and team members is essential. Educate the dancer to talk about diagnostic test results, activity progression, and new pain or uncertainty with their providers. Encourage dialogue when something is not clear. Many dancers have a higher body awareness compared with other patients or even other athletes, and this communication establishes the dancer as an integral part of the medical team.

Table 1
Dance medicine rehabilitation progression protocol

I: Initial Assessment	II: Injury Treatment	III: Progression	IV: Dance-Specific Movement	V: Return to Rehearsal	VI: Independence
Dance-specific history	Pain management	Range of motion	Turnout	Involve artistic director or teacher	Training regimen
Neuromusculoskeletal examination	Swelling and inflammation management	Flexibility	Balance progression	Dynamic warm-up	Transition to maintenance program
Dance-specific tests and considerations	Support and stabilization	Strengthening	Turn progression	Active recovery and cool down	Continuous monitoring
Mental health	Manual therapy	Motor control/proprioception	Jump progression	Dance-specific environment	
Nutrition	Fitness maintenance	Imagery and somatic practice	Partnering and lifting		
Establish diagnosis and injury specific protocols	Home exercise program				

Adapted from Hrubes M. Return–to-Dance Strategies and Guidelines for the Dancer. In: Elson LE, ed. Performance Arts Medicine. 1st ed. St. Louis, MO: Elsevier; 2019:139–149; with permission.

PHASE I: INITIAL ASSESSMENT

The initial evaluation should include a dance-specific history, neuromusculoskeletal examination with dance-specific tests, and assessment of mental health and nutrition.

DANCE-SPECIFIC HISTORY

Exacerbating and alleviating movements are an important component of the history, and it is recommended to use dance terminology if known or have the dancer demonstrate specific actions. Address activities outside of dance to also inform the rehabilitation schedule. Many dancers are students, teachers, and/or work additional jobs to supplement their income. Consequently, how they use their bodies outside of dance might affect their injury and recovery. Other considerations include past medical and injury history, styles of dance, amount of hours spent dancing per week, and shoe wear.

NEUROMUSCULOSKELETAL EVALUATION

The musculoskeletal examination addresses both neurologic and musculoskeletal components of injury in addition to posture, alignment, joint range of motion, flexibility, strength, and cardioconditioning. Even when the injury seems localized, the musculoskeletal evaluation must be generalized and the practitioner must assess regional interdependence. Frequently, patients will dance injured before realizing that medical intervention is necessary. Sometimes secondary injuries occur, or secondary pain sites develop due to altered arthrokinematics.

Posture and Alignment

Baseline posture varies among dance styles due to aesthetic differences. It is important to evaluate for correct postural muscle activation as well as compensations due to muscle tightness, weakness, or joint hypermobility. The dancer should demonstrate dance-specific positions while the practitioner looks for symmetry between sides and aberrant movement patterns.

Joint Range of Motion

At minimum, the range of motion of the lumbar spine, bilateral hips, knees, ankles, and great toes is assessed. If a dancer is trained in classical ballet, passive hip external range of motion is compared with total active turnout.[7] Classical ballet turnout is well researched, but debate continues on the determinants of range of motion and how it should be measured. Dance style will determine how much range of motion is necessary at each joint, and loss of range of motion at one joint leads to increased stress at an adjacent joint. One way to measure functional plantar flexion of the dancer's ankle is the Novella test (**Fig. 1**), which assesses angular deviation between the medial sagittal surfaces of the talar neck/navicular and the distal third of the tibia while the foot is in maximum plantar flexion.[8] It has also been suggested to measure functional ankle dorsiflexion with the lunge test.[9]

Flexibility

Asymmetries in flexibility may be an early sign of injury. Dancers tend to be more flexible than nondancers.[10] Inexperience with the unique requirements of dancers may lead to an erroneous conclusion that a dancer has adequate flexibility when it may be inadequate for their needs.

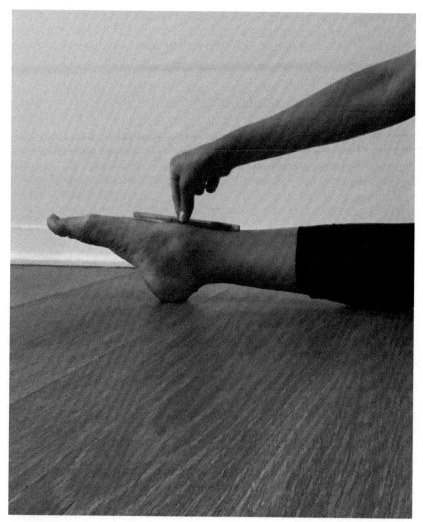

Fig. 1. Novella test.

Strength

The practitioner should use manual muscle tests in the dance-specific ranges of motion. Comparison to the contralateral side is recommended. Isometric manual muscle testing can be more helpful, as isokinetic measurements have indicated lower torque values in dancers than in other athletes, possibly due to ballet dancers having predominately slow twitch fibers.[11] Proper strength is also important in increasing bone health and preventing osteoporosis in dancers.[11]

Cardioconditioning

A dancer's current level of cardioconditioning, such as their weekly cardiovascular routine, should be assessed. Performance demands vary widely[12] depending on the type of dance, choreography, and role, and dancers demonstrate low levels of aerobic fitness even though a strong aerobic foundation is required to meet their workload.[13]

Dance class or rehearsal does not adequately train the dancer for dance performance.[12,14,15] Adequate conditioning[12] decreases the rate of fatigue, and fatigue is associated with increased injury.[16] Common ways to assess a dancer's cardiovascular fitness include Vo_{2Max} test,[17] 3-minute step test,[18] or the dance-specific aerobic fitness test.[19]

DANCE-SPECIFIC TESTS AND CONSIDERATIONS
Joint Hypermobility

Although hypermobility can be an advantage for some dancers, it may increase the risk of injury.[20–22] Hypermobility is associated with an increased injury recovery time when compared with dancers with nonjoint hypermobility syndrome.[23] In addition, benign joint hypermobility syndrome is associated with increased reporting of joint pain.[20] Dancers should be screened for hypermobility using the Beighton Assessment of Hypermobility Scale.[20] If further diagnostic assessment for hypermobility is warranted, the practitioner can use The Lower Limb Assessment Score[24,25] and/or the Upper Limb Hypermobility Assessment Tool.[26]

Balance and Proprioception

A dancer's balance and proprioception are both key to the most fundamental movements of dance, and these can be evaluated in dance-specific positions such as passé (**Fig. 2**) or arabesque (**Fig. 3**). These tests can be tested statically in single limb or double limb balance with eyes open and closed or dynamically with the dancer performing 16 single leg sautés (hops) or the topple test (pirouette in fourth position).[27]

Dance Movements

Dancers who study ballet should have genre-specific evaluation of the biomechanics of common movements. First, ask them to demonstrate first (**Fig. 4**A), second (**Fig. 4**B), fourth (**Fig. 4**C), and fifth (**Fig. 4**D) positions to gain a general understanding of how the dancer moves and have them add in arms to assess scapular movement. Perform plié in each of these positions. There should be even weight-bearing with the calcaneus remaining on the ground throughout the movement. In addition, confirm symmetric turnout and knee flexion aligned over the second toe. Look for improper biomechanics including toe curling, pronation, or anterior tibialis recruitment. Assess spinal mobility with lumbar extension and forward flexion ("cambre" and "port de bras"), monitoring for segmental movement without hinging at a specific level, or excessive lateral lean or rotation. Observe the dancer from the front and side as they jump to ensure their knees, hips, and core contribute to movement and their heels make contact with the floor in a controlled manner. Improper mechanics include lumbar hyperlordosis or landing without a forefoot to heel control. For single leg hop, the pelvis should not drop and the knee should avoid a valgus moment. An injury may preclude a dancer from participating in the full examination.

Turnout

Functional turnout should be assessed by looking for signs of forced turnout, such as increased anterior pelvic tilt, "screwing" the knees with excessive external tibial rotation, or subtalar joint excessive pronation (**Fig. 5**). Traditionally, the range of motion necessary for proper turnout has been accepted as 70° from the femoral-acetabular joint[28]; however, many recent studies have suggested the actual range of motion of the typical ballet dancer hip is between 39.7 and 52.0°.[29–31] This suggests there is more range of motion obtained than the traditional understanding of 5° from the tibial external rotation at the knee and 15° from the ankle and foot. Tools to assist in proper

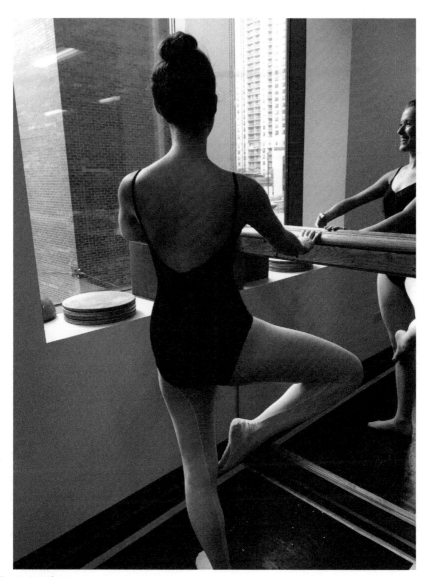

Fig. 2. Passé.

measurement of active and passive range of motion include a goniometer, rotator discs (**Fig. 6**), or functional footprints.

MENTAL HEALTH

Psychological variables are known to affect the outcome of dance injuries in both student and professional dancers.[32] Times of stress, such as an injury, can exacerbate preexisting mental health conditions or prolong the length of recovery.[33] These symptoms might not have surfaced during the initial injury but may come to light with the mental and physical challenges of rehabilitation. The level of fear a dancer experiences

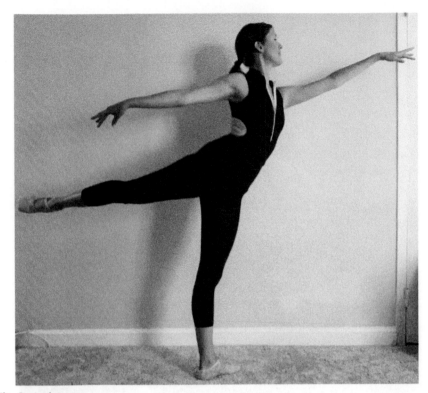

Fig. 3. Arabesque.

after an injury is consistently associated with poor injury recovery outcomes and should be addressed throughout the recovery and rehabilitation process.[34] For professional dancers, an injury increases the likelihood of losing a company position.[35]

Mental fatigue is also of concern for dancers. Understanding the influence psychological factors have on the injured dancer, and encouraging the dancer to address them, can positively affect the duration and outcome of injury rehabilitation.[36,37]

NUTRITION

Evaluating for restricted eating or an eating disorder is important. Dancers are more likely to have a history of an eating disorder than the general population.[38] Nutrition needs to be optimized for recovery from any injury. If there is low bone mineral density, fatigue due to inadequate energy intake, or anemia contributed to the injury, involve a nutritionist/registered dietician. If inadequate energy intake was intentional, then also involve a psychologist and/or psychiatrist.

ESTABLISH DIAGNOSIS AND INJURY-SPECIFIC PROTOCOLS

Once an appropriate history, physical examination, and review of previous management of the injury have been completed, an accurate diagnosis should be made. Even if a definitive diagnosis cannot be made without further diagnostic testing, establish the mechanism of injury if known. Communicate any restrictions or progression

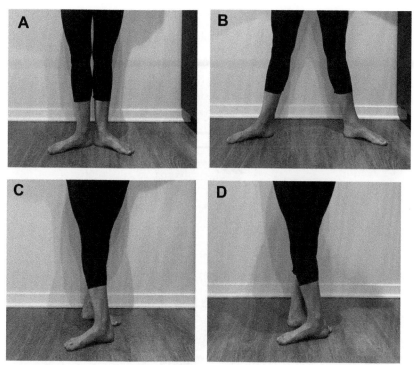

Fig. 4. (*A*) First position. (*B*) Second position. (*C*) Fourth position. (*D*) Fifth position.

protocols, such as weight-bearing in a stress fracture or directional preference in a spine injury.

PHASE II: INJURY MANAGEMENT

After the initial assessment, focus shifts to managing early injury symptoms of pain, swelling and inflammation, and protection of the injury. This phase also includes manual therapy, maintaining fitness, and home exercise program.

Pain Management

Dancer comfort is priority in rehabilitation. If necessary, medications should be used, with clear expectations. Pain medications may be taken, as needed, with consideration of a dancer's medical condition or other medications. Sometimes, a nonsteroidal antiinflammatory drug is given at a high dose to prevent heterotopic ossification or is avoided to promote inflammatory response. The reasoning for prescribing or withholding medications should be made clear to the dancer, including the use of supplements or over-the-counter medications. Many dancers prefer "complementary" medications or treatments, and this should be discussed with the treatment plan. Although pain medications might be necessary early in an injury, they must be stopped before initiating return to dance. Pain or discomfort provides important warning signals and allows minor issues to be addressed as part of the rehabilitation process.

Modalities such as thermal modalities, ultrasound, phonophoresis, and/or electrotherapy provide options for pain management.

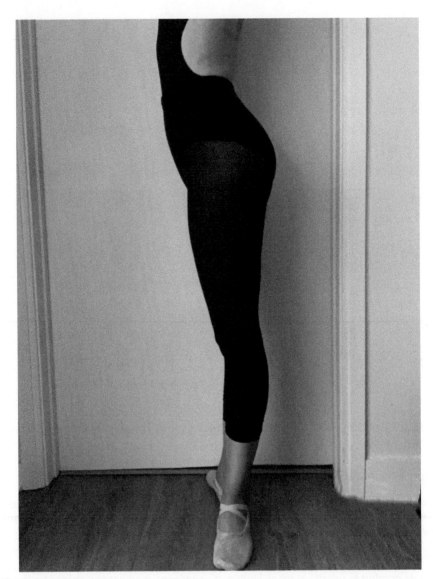

Fig. 5. Forced turnout.

Swelling and Inflammation Management

Swelling is common after injury and can lead to muscle inhibition with slow rehabilitation progression. An ankle joint effusion decreases peroneus longus activity,[39] and 20 mL of excess fluid in the knee joint causes arthrogenic inhibition of the vastus medialis muscle.[40] Compression can reduce posttraumatic edema, inflammatory response, and soft tissue scarring while improving proprioceptive feedback[41]; this can be done with taping, wrapping, bracing, or intermittent pneumatic compression. A short course of antiinflammatory medication may be appropriate if swelling limits range of motion or causes compensatory movement patterns. When using

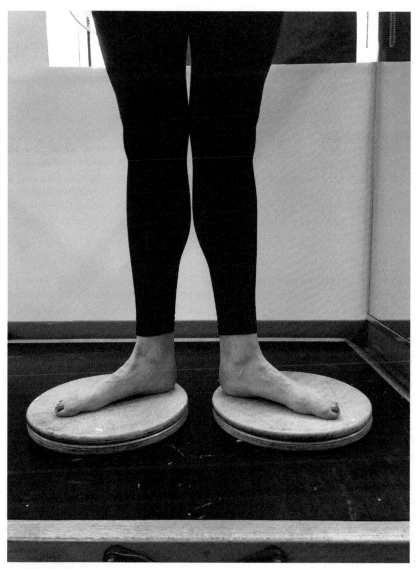

Fig. 6. Rotator discs.

antiinflammatory medication, consider a purposeful approach, such as a prescription strength dose, with a 1-week time limit.

Support and Stabilization

Support for injured muscles, ligaments, and joints is important to prevent further injury and compensatory behaviors. Stabilization should be prioritized after a ligament tear, joint subluxation, or dislocation and can be specifically helpful in dancers with hypermobility. If the dancer is able to perform during the rehabilitation process, bracing is often not possible due to aesthetics. Taping is less bulky and commonly used, with 27.6% of surveyed dance medicine physical therapists[42] using many tape types for injured dancers. Taping can be used for support and stability,[43] compression, proprioception,[44] facilitation of muscle concentric contraction,[45] promotion of muscle inhibition in hypertonic muscles,[46] or even to promote dancer confidence.[47] Orthotics can also be used to promote proper biomechanics, particularly with hyperpronation,[48] and can be modified to fit ballet slippers or stage shoes.

Manual Therapy

Manual therapy should be used to mobilize soft tissue, improve joint motion, and decrease edema. After injury, tissue mobilization is necessary to avoid scarring, contractures, and muscle inhibition. Muscle tightness may be in response to joint instability, so use caution releasing muscle, as it could lead to injury recurrence. Joint contracture can occur after prolonged immobilization. Joint malalignment may be premorbid or in response to injury. Manual therapy can include myofascial release with hands or tools, joint mobilization or manipulation, massage, or manual traction. Additional manual therapy options include dry needling, trigger point injections, acupuncture, and cupping.

Fitness Maintenance

It is important to keep an injured dancer moving to preserve cardiovascular fitness and avoid deconditioning and atrophy. Provide the injured dancer with modified or alternative activities that are safe to perform. This also offers the dancer an alternative outlet for their energy and time. When possible, integrate dance participation early into the rehabilitation plan, creating space to maintain their dancer identity. Modified dance class may include work at the barre without moving to center, keeping extension low, avoiding jumps, and/or restricting activity to the noninjured limb. When regular dance class participation is not safe, consider Floor Barre, Aqua Barre, Pilates, and/or Gyrotonic with modifications to accommodate injury restrictions.

If injury is due to or concurrent with disordered eating or relative energy deficiency in sport, careful consideration of energy availability and its relation to bone and cardiac health is vital before integrating cardiovascular maintenance into the rehabilitation process.

Home Exercise Program

Starting a home exercise program early in the rehabilitation process establishes it as an important and integral part of return to dance. Initial exercises can focus on preserving joint range of motion and muscle activation. Although some dancers might not be compliant with the home exercises assigned, others might do the program in excess, which can also be counterproductive. Understanding why the rehabilitation is important helps the dancer find motivation and gain perspective on the process.[42]

PHASE III: PROGRESSION

During this phase, deficits found during initial assessment including range of motion, flexibility, strengthening, motor control/proprioception, and imagery and somatic practice are addressed. A solid foundation for rehabilitation is established and previous modifications are adjusted.

Range of Motion

Dancers are significantly more likely to change their level of dance if they return after injury with a decreased or limited range of motion.[34] Restricted posterior glide of the talocrural joint occurs even when dorsiflexion has been restored after an ankle sprain.[49] Educate dancers on safe joint range of motion, as their sensation of a muscle stretch can be affected by generalized ligamentous laxity or previous injury.

Flexibility

Flexibility is crucial in many styles of dance and is a product of muscle extensibility and joint mobility,[50] so stretching is fundamental to dancers. Stretching increases tendon unit compliance, increasing the amount of energy absorbed by the tendon when the muscle is activated, which reduces muscle fiber trauma.[51] In dance, this is beneficial for jump landing, which elongates the Achilles immediately after the gastrosoleus complex concentrically contracts to initiate the jump.

There are many types of stretches, with various benefits or risk of injury. Proprioceptive neuromuscular facilitation (PNF) is a more effective form of stretching than static or ballistic[52] and also improves muscle strength after 8 weeks.[53] It has been found that a combination of static and PNF stretching improved postexercise flexibility of the hip adductors in female ballet dancers.[54] Thirty seconds of static stretching is more effective than a shorter duration and as effective as holding a stretch for a longer period of time.[55] Static stretching should not be the sole warm-up stretch before class, rehearsal, or performance, as it reduces muscle strength at slow contraction velocities for the next 1 to 2 hours.[56] One survey of ballet students (aged 17–25 years) found that 88% of rear thigh injuries occurred during slow activities such as flexibility training with splits in sagittal plane or warm-up/cool down, whereas only 12% of the injuries occurred during powerful movements such as large jumps.[57]

Strengthening

Strengthening should address preinjury weakness and/or weakness that developed after injury. Dancers might not have true neurologic weakness, and instead have strength mismatch,[58] causing maladaptive compensation techniques. Perceived loss of strength by the dancer is associated with significantly increased recovery time,[34] and strength imbalances increase injury risk.[59]

Initiate strengthening with controlled, isolated movements to minimize compensation by other muscles, providing neuromuscular reeducation when necessary to encourage proper form and movement patterns. Movements should be broken down and retrained to ensure correct biomechanics. Begin with isometric movements, progressing to isotonic, and then isokinetic as appropriate.[41] The overload principle is important in order to stimulate muscle change.[11] Then, create strengthening exercises using dance-specific movements and increase movement complexity with a goal of integrating the activation of multiple muscles at an increasing tempo in dance movement patterns.

Reassure the injured dancer that muscle strength can be gained without increased muscle bulk or loss of flexibility.[11] Some dancers avoid strength training under the impression that their muscles will hypertrophy, which they may perceive as negatively affecting their aesthetic appearance.[11] Others avoid strength training due to concern for loss of flexibility, when in fact strength training is positively associated with flexibility scores.[11,60]

Motor Control/Proprioception

Motor control after injury is important. Proper control is a combination of neural (proprioception, reflexes, muscular reaction time), muscular (strength, power, and endurance), and mechanical (ligaments) factors.[61]

As ligaments are integral to structural stability, proprioceptive training is of particular importance for dancers with hypermobility. Postural stability of classical ballet dancers was impaired for several weeks after ankle sprain when comparing their pre-injury with postinjury postural sway, which improved with rehabilitation.[62] The dancer needs to understand hip/pelvis disassociation, scapular placement, and maintaining a neutral spine and pelvis as a foundation for the progression of dance-specific mechanics. Emphasize deep core control, isometric cocontraction when appropriate, and eccentric stabilization, especially at end range of motion. Initiate proprioceptive training with weight shifting, and then single leg balance on a stable surface, progressing to an unstable surface. Neuromuscular reeducation provides a dynamically stable joint that improves function and reduces reinjury risk.[63]

Imagery and Somatic Practice

Imagery and somatic practice can be introduced as methods to improve motor learning.[64] Imagery, or visualizing movement, enhances coping skills of injured athletes and promotes rehabilitation adherence.[65] Mental imagery focusing on healing and relaxation is associated with improved pain tolerance.[66] Somatic practices such as the Feldenkrais Method for mindful movement or Alexander Technique improve awareness of movement patterns.

PHASE IV: DANCE-SPECIFIC MOVEMENT

When the injury has healed and a firm foundation for recovery is in place, progression to more complex maneuvers is appropriate to prepare the dancer for return to class, rehearsal, and performances. When progressing through increasingly difficult physical demands, remind the dancers to listen to their body and proceed in a step-wise fashion. Delayed pain can be an indication of progression that is advancing too quickly. Soreness can be a positive indication that muscles are appropriately challenged. This can be an opportunity to dialogue with the dancer on knowing differences between pain and soreness, in order to prevent future injuries.

Regular status checks are critical to assess progress, goal achievement, estimated return to dance, and modifications when necessary. To help keep the dancer focused, there may be adjustments to home exercises, correction of previous assumptions, and reminders of overall goals.

Turnout

Turnout is an important foundation to many dance-specific movements. Any discrepancy between total passive turnout and total active turnout should be addressed. Muscle weakness or tightness, tissue restriction, and poor motor control[67] can lead to forced turnout. Note that a dancer's turnout is typically not symmetric between legs, so often education to minimize cheating on the less mobile leg is necessary. Dancers can improve active turnout by strengthening the hip external rotators.[68,69]

Balance Progression

Once the dancer has established baseline motor control and proprioception, they can progress to balance in dance-specific movements. This can include static positions in addition to dynamic challenges, such as single leg stance with gesture leg movement. The dancer will then progress to traveling combinations to include dynamic balance and relearning to stop in a combination for a static hold. An example of balance progression would be changing from linear or angular movement, changing dance shoes, adding distractions as experienced on stage, adding props/costumes, or changing movement tempo with a metronome.

Turn Progression

When it is appropriate to integrate turns, start with turn preparation from a wide to a narrow base of support ("fourth" to "fifth" position). This ensures that the dancer can begin turning upright from a strong foundation in proper position from both feet. Progress from single turns, to multiple turns, and then traveling turns. Have the dancer use different dance shoes, eventually progressing to pointe shoes if applicable. In addition challenge the dancer by changing arm variations, leg extensions, levels, combinations, adding props/costumes, changing tempo with music, and adding distractions.

Jump Progression

Jumping requires endurance, range of motion, proprioception, and strength. Classical ballet dancers perform more than 200 jumps per 1.5-hour daily technique class,[70] yet suffer considerably fewer anterior cruciate ligament injuries than athletes participating in team ball sports.[71] Jumping should start with repetitive releves, focusing on controlled mechanics. The dancer will need to focus on alignment, equal weight distribution, core control, relaxed shoulders, and controlled landing to the heel. The dancer should then progress to double leg jumping in basic first or second positions in both parallel and turnout, moving to more challenging positions such as fifth position. Once the dancer can execute double leg jumping with control and proper technique, then single leg hopping in place can be performed in both parallel and turnout. They can then progress to low-traveling weight shifts across the floor and then to higher-level explosive jumps. Challenges should be incorporated, including changing shoes, adding costumes and props, changing tempo, changing from linear to angular movements such as a jump turn, adding jump combinations, and increasing repetitions. Continue to monitor symptoms while progressing to adjust load or jump frequency if inflammation or pain occurs.

Partnering and Lifting

Throughout rehabilitation, be aware of the partner's lift expectations. Have the partner attend sessions to address typical lifts. Dancers should attempt their lifts in costume when ready to address any safety concerns. Review choreography and address any challenges with the dancer and artistic staff.

PHASE V: RETURN TO REHEARSAL

When returning to full participation in class and rehearsal, continue formal rehabilitation to address any difficulties or concerns that arise, working toward full mastery of the skills.

Involve Artistic Director or Teacher

With the dancer's permission, communicate with the dancer's artistic director, staff, or teacher throughout rehabilitation as appropriate. They may be essential to successful transition, particularly after a prolonged absence or when the company/studio does not have in-house medical staff. During this phase, ask if they will take the dancer through a modified class, as they often identify areas of concern that might limit the dancer's return, from technique to aesthetics or anxiety. Staff is also aware of upcoming choreography styles and demands, allowing the dancer to better prepare physically and mentally.

Dynamic Warm-Up

Educate the dancer on the importance of preparing the mind and body for class, rehearsal, and performance. A light cardiovascular warm-up such as walking, marching, body swing, and step-hops around the room, followed by 30 seconds of static stretches then 30 seconds of dynamic stretches can improve balance, jump height, and hamstring range of motion in female ballet dancers.[72] Encourage easy movement of the ankles, knees, hips, and shoulders to activate muscles and gradually increase heart rate and body temperature. Discourage aggressive static stretching or over-stretching as it can increase injury risk[73] and lead to muscle inhibition.[56] Tailor the warm-up to address areas of tightness or muscles the dancer has difficulty activating and consider performance-specific choreography such as leaps or turns.

Active Recovery and Cool Down

The cool down allows for gradual decrease in body temperature and heart rate and is the appropriate time for soft tissue stretching and mobilization with foam rolling, hand held rollers, and massage balls. Depending on resources available, cryotherapy or compression boots can assist with recovery. Nutrition can play a role in recovery as well; and early rehydration with an appropriate fluid can improve the athlete's endurance and total work performed in the next exercise session by improving muscle glycogen replenishment.[74]

Dance-Specific Environment

Simulate the environment as much as possible, including flooring material such as a sprung floor, wood slats, steel, or tile. Stages can be raked (at an incline) or flat; consequently it may be appropriate to perform some of the rehabilitation on a raked surface. Footwear type, such a tap shoes, pointe shoes, or ghillies in Irish dance, greatly affect the way a dancer interacts with the floor. The rehabilitation practitioner should ensure good fit and biomechanics when the dancer is in footwear. Costumes that involve heavy headdresses or restrictive corsets change the center of gravity and breathing technique. These may be used during practice. Dancers must concentrate despite bright or flashing lights, audience chatter, and other performers. Face the dancer away from the mirror so they do not rely on watching themselves for technique or balance. Vary lighting, using a bright light to simulate a spotlight, or require eyes closed to simulate when all lights are turned off onstage ("blackout").

PHASE VI: INDEPENDENCE

When formal rehabilitation is complete, and the dancer has successfully returned to their previous level of function, the dancer is not finished but has transitioned to an independent maintenance program. This program is integrated into warm-up, class, rehearsals, and performances, with the goal of minimizing reinjury and preventing new injury. In cases of prolonged recovery, consider scheduling a reassessment a few weeks after promotion to self-sufficiency. This provides opportunity to address any pain or dysfunction that may arise, correct exercise biomechanics, revisit issues the dancer struggled with throughout rehab, address new choreography concerns, and adjust the maintenance plan accordingly.

DISCLOSURE

The authors have nothing to disclose.

REFERENCES

1. Ojofeitimi S, Bronner S. Injuries in a modern dance company: effect of comprehensive management on injury incidence and cost. J Dance Med Sci 2011;15:
   116–22.
2. Ekegren C, Quested R, Brodnick A. Injuries in pre-professional ballet dancers:
   incidence, characteristics and consequences. J Sci Med Sport 2014;17:271–5.
3. Kenny SJ, Whittaker JL, Emery CA. Risk factors for musculoskeletal injury in pre-
   professional dancers: a systematic review. Br J Sports Med 2015;0:1–8.
4. Solomon R, Micheli L, Solomon J, et al. The "cost" of injuries in a professional
   ballet company: anatomy of a season. Med Probl Perform Artists 1995;
   10(1):3–10.
5. Hrubes M. Return-to-dance strategies and guidelines for the dancer. In: Elston L,
   editor. Performing arts medicine. St Louis (MO): Elsevier; 2019. p. 140.
6. Anakwe R, Jenkins P, Moran M. Predicting dissatisfaction after total hip arthroplasty: a study of 850 patients. J Arthroplasty 2011;26:209–13.
7. Liederbach M. Screening for functional capacity in dancers. J Dance Med Sci
   1997;1:93–106.
8. Novella TM. Simple techniques for quantifying choreographically essential foot
   and ankle extents of motion. J Dance Med Sci 2004;8(4):118–22.
9. Dickson D, Hollman-Gage K, Ojofeitimi S, et al. Comparison of functional ankle
   motion measures in modern dancers. J Dance Med Sci 2012;16(3):116–25.
10. DiTullio M, Wilczek L, Paulus D, et al. Comparison of hip rotation in female clas-
    sical ballet dancers versus female nondancers. Med Probl Perform Art 1999;4:
    154–8.
11. Koutedakis Y, Stravropoulos-Kalinoglou A, Metsios G. The significance of
    muscular strength in dance. J Dance Med Sci 2005;9(1):29–34.
12. Wyon M. Cardiorespiratory training for dancers. J Dance Med Sci 2005;9:7–12.
13. Twitchett EA, Koutedakis Y, Wyon MA. Physiological fitness and professional clas-
    sical ballet performance: a brief review. J Strength Cond Res 2009;23(9):
    2732–40.
14. Cohen J, Segal K, McARdle W. Heart rate response to ballet state performance.
    Pys Sportsmed 1982;10:120–33.
15. Schantz P, Astrand P. Physiologic characteristics of classical ballet. Med Sci
    Sports Exerc 1984;16:472–6.
16. Liederbach M, Gleim GW, Nichols JA. Physiologic and psychosocial measure-
    ments of performance stress and onset of injuries in professional ballet dancers.
    Med Probl Perform Art 1994;9(1):10–4.
17. Wyon MA, Allen N, Cloak R, et al. Assessment of maximum aerobic capacity and
    anaerobic threshold of elite ballet dancers. Med Probl Perform Art 2016;31(3):
    145–50.
18. Bronner S, Ojofeitimi S, Lora JB, et al. A preseason cardiorespiratory profile of
    dancers in nine professional ballet and modern companies. J Dance Med Sci
    2014;18(2):74–85.
19. Wyon M, Redding E, Abt G, et al. Development, reliability, validity of a multistage
    dance specific aerobic fitness test (DAFT). J Dance Med Sci 2003;7(3):80–4.
20. McCormack M, Briggs J, Hakim A, et al. Joint laxity and the benign joint hyper-
    mobility syndrome in student and professional ballet dancers. J Rheumatol
    2004;31:173–8.
21. Hamilton W, Hamilton L, Marshall P. A profile of the musculoskeletal characteris-
    tics of elite professional ballet dancers. Am J Sports Med 1992;20:267–73.

22. Micheli L, Gillespie W, Walaszek A. Physiologic profiles of female professional ballerinas. Clin Sports Med 1984;3:199–209.
23. Briggs J, McCormack M, Hakim A, et al. Injury and joint hypermobility syndrome in ballet dancers – a 5-year follow-up. J Rheumatol 2009;48:1613–4.
24. Ferrari J, Parslow C, Lim E, et al. Andrew. Joint hypermobility: the use of a new assessment tool to measure lower limb hypermobility. Clin Exp Rheumatol 2005;23(3):413–20.
25. Meyer KJ, Chan C, Hopper L, et al. Identifying lower limb specific and general-ized joint hypermobility in adults: validation of lower limb assessment score. BMC Musculoskelet Disord 2017;18:514, 1-9.
26. Nicholson L, Chan C. The upper limb hypermobility assessment tool: A novel vali-dated measure of adult joint mobility. Musculoskelet Sci Pract 2018;35:38–45.
27. Richardson M, Liederbach M, Sandow E. Functional criteria for assessing pointe readiness. J Dance Med Sci 2015;6(1):6–7.
28. Thomasen E. Diseases and injuries of ballet dancers. Arjus (Denmark): Arhus Universitetsforlaget I; 1982 (English translation).
29. Bauman P, Singson R, Hamilton W. Femoral neck anteversion in ballerinas. Clin Orthop 1994;(302):57–63.
30. Gilbert C, Gross M, Klug K. Relationship between hip external rotation and turnout angle for the five classical ballet positions. J Orthop Sports Phys Ther 1998;27:339–47.
31. Khan K, Roberts P, Nattrass C, et al. Hip and ankle range of motion in elite clas-sical ballet dancer and controls. Clin J Sport Med 1997;7:174–9.
32. Mainwaring L, Finney C. Psychological risk factors and outcomes of dance injury, a systematic review. J Dance Med Sci 2017;21:87–96.
33. Thomas J, Keel P, Heatherton T. Disordered eating and injuries among adoles-cent ballet dancers. Eat Weight Disord 2011;16:e216–22.
34. Junck E, Richardson M, Dilgen F, et al. A retrospective assessment of return to function in dance after physical therapy for common dance injuries. J Dance Med Sci 2017;21:156–67.
35. Garrick J, Requa R. Ballet injuries: an analysis of epidemiological and financial outcome. Am J Sports Med 1993;12:586–90.
36. Mainwaring L, Krasnow D, Kerr G. And the dance goes on: psychological impact of injury. J Dance Med Sci 2001;5:105–15.
37. Noh Y, Morris T, Anderses M. Psychological intervention programs for reduction of injury in ballet dancers. Res Sports Med 2007;15:13–32.
38. Arcelus J, Witcomb G, Mitchell A. Prevalence of eating disorders amongst dancers: a systemic review and meta-analysis. Eur Eat Disord Rev 2014;22(2):92–101.
39. Hopkin J, Palmieri R. Effects of ankle joint effusion on lower leg function. Clin J Sport Med 2004;14:1–7.
40. Spencer J, Hayes K, Alexancer I. Knee joint effusion and quadriceps reflex inhi-bition in man. Arch Phys Med Rehabil 1984;65:171–7.
41. Clanton T, Coupe K. Hamstring strains in athletes: diagnosis and treatment. J Am Acad Orthop Surg 1998;6:237–48.
42. Sabo M. Physical therapy rehabilitation strategies for dancers: a qualitative study. J Dance Med Sci 2013;17:11–7.
43. Ewalt K. Bandaging and taping considerations of the dancer. J Dance Med Sci 2010;14:103–13.

44. Cools A, Witvrouw E, Danneels L, et al. Does taping influence electromyographic muscle activity in the scapular rotators in healthy shoulders? Man Ther 2002;7: 154–62.
45. Thelen M, Dauber J, Stoneman P. The clinical efficacy of kinsio tape for shoulder pain: a randomized, double-blinded, clinical trial. J Orthop Sports Phys Ther 2008;38:389–95.
46. Yasukawa A, Patel P, Sisung C. Pilot study: investigating the effects of Kinesio Taping in an acute pediatric rehabilitation setting. Am J Occup Ther 2006;60: 104–10.
47. Sawkins K, Refsuage K, Kilbreath S, et al. The placebo effect of ankle taping in ankle instability. Med Sci Sport Exerc 2007;39:781–7.
48. Nowacki R, Air M, Rietveld A. Use and effectiveness of orthotics in hyperpronated dancers. J Dance Med Sci 2013;17:3–10.
49. Denegar DR, Hertel J, Fonseca J. The effect of lateral ankle sprain on dorsiflexion range of motion, posterior talar glide, and joint laxity. J Orthop Sports Phys Ther 2002;32(4):166–73.
50. Deighan M. Flexibility in dance. J Dance Med Sci 2005;9:13–7.
51. Witvrouw E, Mahieu N, Danneels L, et al. Stretching and injury prevention: an obscure relationship. Sports Med 2005;34:443–9.
52. Sady S, Wortman M, Blanke D. Flexibility training: ballistic, static or proprioceptive neuromuscular facilitation. Arch Phys Med Rehabil 1982;63:261–3.
53. Handel M, Horstmann T, Dickhutch H, et al. Effects of contract-relax stretching training on muscle performance in athetes. Eur J Appl Physiol 1997;76:400–8.
54. Rubini E, Souza A, Mello M, et al. Immediate effect of static and proprioceptive neuromuscular facilitation stretching on hip adductor flexibility in female ballet dancers. J Dance Med Sci 2011;15(4):177–81.
55. Roberts J, Wilson K. Effect of stretching duration on the active and passive range of motion in the lower extremity. Br J Sports Med 1999;33:259–63.
56. Power K, Behm D, Cahill F, et al. An acute bout of staic stretching: Effects of force and jumping performance. Med Sci Sports Exerc 2004;36:1389–96.
57. Askling C, Lund H, Saartok T, et al. Self-reported hamstring injuries in student dancers. Scand J Me Sci Sports 2002;12:230–5.
58. Liederbach M, Hiebert R. The relationship between eccentric and concentric equinus in classical dancers. J Dance Med Sci 1997;1:55–61.
59. Aagaard P, Simonsen E, Magnusson S, et al. A new concept for isokinetic hamstring: Quadriceps muscle strength ratio. Am J Sports Med 1998;26:231–7.
60. Pratt M. Strength, flexibility, and maturity in adolescent athletes. Am J Dis Child 1989;143:560–3.
61. Konradsen L, Olesen S, Hansen H. Ankle sensorimotor control and eversion strength after acute ankle inversion injuries. Am J Sports Med 1998;26:72–7.
62. Leanderson J, Eriksson E, Nilsson C, et al. Proprioception in classical ballet dancers. A prospective study of the influence of an ankle sprain on proprioception in the ankle joint. Am J Sports Med 1996;24(3):370–4.
63. Griffin L, Agel J, Albohm M, et al. Noncontact anterior cruciate ligament injuries: Risk factors and prevention strategies. J Am Acad Orthop Surg 2000;8:141–50.
64. Baston G. Revisiting overuse injuries in dance in view of motor learning and somatic models of distributed practice. J Dance Med Sci 2007;11:70–5.
65. Wesch N, Hall C, Prapavessis H, et al. Self-efficacy, imagery use, and adherence during injury rehabilitation. Scand J Med Sci Sports 2012;22:695–703.

66. Hamson-Utley J, Martin S, Walters J. Athletic trainer's and physical therapists' perceptions of the effectiveness of psychological skills within sport injury rehabilitation programs. J Athl Train 2008;43:258–64.
67. Grossman G. Measuring dancer's active and passive turnout. J Dance Med Sci 2003;7:49–55.
68. Pata D, Welsh T, Bailey J, et al. Improving turnout in university dancers. J Dance Med Sci 2014;18:169–77.
69. Sherman AJ, Mayall E, Tasker SL. Can a prescribed turnout conditioning program reduce the differential between passive and active turnout in pre-professional dancers? J Dance Med Sci 2014;18(4):159–68.
70. Liederbach M, Richardson M, Rodriguez M, et al. Jump exposures in the dance training environment: a measure of ergonomic demand. J Athl Train 2006; 41(2):S85.
71. Liederbach M, Dilgen F, Rose D. Incidence of anterior cruciate ligament injuries among elite ballet and modern dancers: a 5-year prospective study. Am J Sports Med 2008;36(9):1779–88.
72. Morrin N, Redding E. Acute effects of warm-up stretch protocols on balance, vertical jump height, and range of motion in dancers. J Dance Med Sci 2013;17: 34–40.
73. Shrier I. When and whom to stretch? Gauging the benefits and drawbacks for individual patients. Physician Sports Med 2004;33:22–6.
74. Karp RJ, Johnston JD, Tecklenburg S, et al. Chocolate milk as a post-exercise recovery aid. Int J Sport Nutr Exerc 2006;16(1):78–91.

Access to Health Care Among Dancers

Carolyn E. Keeler, DO

KEYWORDS

- Dancer • Injury • Access • Health care • Prevention

KEY POINTS

- Dancers are a subset of athletes with unique health care considerations that require specialized care.
- Dancers' perceptions of the health care system affect their decision to seek care, choice of provider, and use of ancillary services.
- There are potential deficits in health care for dancers, including access to primary care, financial burden of accessing care, and availability of services.
- Efforts to close gaps in care are ongoing, with an expanding number of health care professionals developing expertise in the care of dancers, continuing education opportunities, community outreach, and professional volunteerism.
- Professional societies dedicated to the promotion of dancer health have seen expansion of membership and offer symposiums for exchange of knowledge to benefit the dance community.

INTRODUCTION/BACKGROUND

Dancers are a subset of athletes with a high injury rate and who rely on specialized health care for recovery and return to performance.[1–15] Dancers receive less public recognition of the physical and mental demands of their art form, and commonly lack the level of financial security that many other professional athletes enjoy. Similar to other athletes, injury rates are significant, with a high annual injury incidence and lifetime prevalence,[1,4,6–8,10–15] with costs of injury in some professional companies being comparable with college athletics and professional sports teams.[6] Most dance injuries are chronic and related to overuse/repetitive microtrauma, with the lower extremity most commonly affected, followed by the lumbar spine.[1,2,5] Overuse injuries are more common than traumatic injuries among amateur and professional dancers, with overuse injuries being more prevalent in amateur ballet dancers, although male professionals have a higher proportion of traumatic injuries.[12,14]

Department of Neurosurgery, Duke University Medical Center, DUMC Box 3807, Durham, NC 27710, USA
E-mail address: carolyn.keeler@duke.edu

Phys Med Rehabil Clin N Am 32 (2021) 21–33
https://doi.org/10.1016/j.pmr.2020.08.004
1047-9651/21/© 2020 Elsevier Inc. All rights reserved.

In treating dancers, it is essential to understand the particular dance genre and injury patterns associated with the various styles. Each dance genre has its own terminology related to technique, and there is variability in the environment in which they train and perform, in addition to different styles of footwear and variations in injury patterns.[3] Dance injury data are most prolific in ballet and modern/contemporary dance. There is a growing body of research into injuries of other dance genres, including jazz, tap, hip-hop, ballroom, and Irish dance; however, epidemiologic data primarily represent ballet and contemporary dance.

It is important for dance medicine clinicians and researchers to understand the historical lack of consistency in methodology for collecting injury data, including defining an injury, exposure information, and details about methodology that would allow reproducibility of research. The dance medicine community has made efforts over the years to build consensus and establish protocols for injury reporting, with the long-term goal of improving efforts toward risk reduction and injury prevention.[16] In considering dance injury research, clinicians should be aware of the variation in definition of a dance injury as time loss, requiring medical attention, or as defined by the dancers' experience, which may vary widely.[17] It is also essential to acknowledge the presence of pain, because dancers may ignore onset of pain as a result of tissue damage, continue to dance despite pain, and not seek care to address the symptoms, which reduces the possibility of early intervention and secondary prevention.[18]

PSYCHOLOGICAL ASPECTS OF INJURY

In order to support dancer health, physicians should acknowledge how fear and stigma surrounding injury play a role while being aware of the potential of delay in reporting and seeking care.[2,19] Dancers' perceptions of injury and pain factor into their decisions to seek care; they may have concerns with accessing the health care system, including feeling poorly understood because of their niche within the athletic population. Negative perception often leads to delay in seeking needed treatment of injury while concurrently driving individuals to continue dancing despite pain and injury.[18] Historically, there has been uneasiness among dancers that seeing a health care professional could result in being told not to dance.[4,20,21] The consequential inability to perform may lead to truncation of career, loss of identity, and psychological distress.[19]

Comorbid psychological stress in injured dancers should be acknowledged, and, in fulfilling the needs of dancers seeking care for an injury, a holistic approach should be considered. Delivery of optimal care is contingent on the understanding of biopsychosocial aspects of dancers. Because formal dance training frequently begins at a young age,[5] dancers develop an identity as a dancer in adolescence. Pain coping styles can affect the physical and psychological health of dancers and should be acknowledged by health care professionals. Personality traits, including perfectionism and the syndrome of the overachiever, can be associated with physical stress and dance injury.[22]

In a study of professional ballet and contemporary dancers, a perception of pain being threatening can indicate nonhelpful coping styles of avoidance and catastrophizing,[23] which has implications of injury chronicity and poorer psychological health. In ballet, despite improvement in rehabilitation and conditioning methods and increased athleticism of the dancers, there is an expectation of injury occurrence during the span of a career. An individual's identity as a dancer is solidified and under threat of a career-ending injury.[24] In a study of amateur and professional dancers in the Netherlands investigating the presence of psychological symptoms coexisting with musculoskeletal injuries, 60% of dancers met the clinical criteria for referral to a psychiatrist or psychologist.[25] When evaluating an injured dancer, clinicians should be aware of the potential for psychological distress and should consider the dancer's possible need for additional psychological support.

Moreover, the psychological well-being of dancers may be negatively affected by the additional stigma surrounding mental health and fear of possible consequences of reporting an injury.[19] Dance educators, choreographers, and company directors are on the front lines of injury and have the ability to partner with health care professionals to support the well-being of dancers. Multiple barriers exist that affect dancers' ability to obtain timely and quality care, including, but not limited to, cost of services, availability of providers with specialized expertise in dance medicine, lack of on-site care, absence of guidance for navigating the health care system, and few systems providing triage of dancers to avoid potential delays in injury management. The availability of high-quality primary and specialty care is essential to meet the needs of the dance community.

PERCEPTIONS HELD BY DANCERS REGARDING PAIN AND INJURY

It is helpful for clinicians to understand dancers' experiences of injury and pain. Injured dancers are affected by both psychological and social factors that can affect the risk of recurrent and chronic injury. Health care–seeking behaviors in dancers must be understood in order to provide care to improve population health. When interpreting such behaviors, it is necessary to study the various concerns dancers may have with reporting an injury. Dance is known to have a culture of pushing through or hiding an injury (the show must go on). Dancers are frequently apprehensive about reporting injury because of the possibility of losing a role or contract, and experience fear in response to the threat of an injury. Despite the consequences of delayed or absent treatment, dancers often face the difficult choice of hiding or minimizing an injury to avoid the loss of performance opportunity and employment. In a study of Australian professional dancers that queried opinions and actions following a dance injury (defined as a physical problem deriving from stress or other causes to do with performance, rehearsal, training, or other circumstances of dance life that affect the ability to participate fully in normal dance training, performance, or physical activity), more than half of the dancers were fearful of short-term and long-term consequences of an injury. Specific fears, in descending order, included inability to perform role to full capacity, casting and contract concerns, future standing in the industry, losing dance identity, psychological health consequences, reinjury, physical issues outside of dance, judgment from others, hindered ability to learn, pain, and financial concerns. Although dancers reported that they would be unlikely to ignore an injury, they expressed concerns of stigma, repercussions, and the tendency to delay reporting an injury. When asked about actions they would take in response to an injury, 70% to 80% reported they would seek a clinical opinion. Other possible actions included taking their own preventive steps, reporting to employer, and using pain medication.[19] In a survey of professional modern dancers in the United States, dancers reported factors that they thought contributed to their injuries, which included demands of their role, self-pressure to excel, demands from choreographer, pain and fatigue, inadequate warm-up, lifestyle factors (sleep, smoking, diet), floor condition, and stage conditions. Minor factors reported included pressure from other dancers and shoe type.[4] An international cross-sectional survey of professional ballet and modern dancers showed that a significant percentage of dancers did not report their injuries, with 15% of ballet dancers and between 9.1% and 18.2% (and with 1 company a high of 66.7%) not reporting an injury. Reasons for not reporting included injury not affecting work, pain as an inherent aspect of dance, being able to cope with pain, and not wanting to stop dancing.[2]

In a study of dance students and former dancers in the United Kingdom, most (>90%) had experienced an injury, defined as not being able to move normally or dance. Rates did not seem to decrease despite efforts to promote dancer health in dance education and professional companies by educating dancers to avoid the no-pain, no-gain mentality, and dancers were noted to report that they would continue to dance despite having an injury. Dancers were more likely to be aware of injuries as they age and were more likely to engage in prevention efforts. Also noted was the likelihood of underreporting of injury in survey data, because dancers were noted to report the experience of pain that they did not equate with an injury.[18] These findings highlight the importance of improving the work culture of dancers for improved long-term dancer health outcomes. By gaining an understanding of dancers' points of view, health care professionals can attempt to bridge the gap and provide high-quality care, and work to develop systems in which dancers are able to obtain specialized care in a cost-effective manner.

HEALTH CARE–SEEKING DECISIONS MADE BY DANCERS

In a study of dancers in the United Kingdom from various dance genres and levels of advancement, the authors investigated psychological factors of injured dancers, including help-seeking behaviors. It was noted that the most common response to an injury was to report it to someone (teacher or director in 68.5%), and most (82.2%) dancers continued to dance, although many reported dancing more carefully than before being injured (68.1%). The injured dancers were most likely to consult a physical therapist (38.1%), and most reported that they would follow medical recommendations, although 21% did not seek professional help. Other choices of providers included massage therapists (21.4%), and less frequently dancers would consult their primary care physicians or specialists. Note that a subset of dancers reported hiding the injury.[26] Another study of injured dancers in the United Kingdom queried dancers regarding actions following a suspected injury, and dancers were most likely to consult physical therapists, Pilates instructors, and massage therapists. The choice of practitioner was thought to be related to the sample population having access to those most frequently affiliated with vocational schools and dance companies in the United Kingdom. It was also noted that the injured dancers were more likely (>53%) to continue to dance with some modification. Many of the dancers (41%) were likely to take self-treatment actions, including use of analgesics (18%), and fewer ignored (6%) or hid (3%) the injury.[27]

In a study conducted in Canada investigating communication between dancers and medical practitioners, Lai and colleagues[18] queried preprofessional and professional dancers, and also surveyed health professionals, including sports medicine physicians, chiropractors, physical therapists, and massage therapists. Of the dancers who sustained an injury, 32% visited a medical professional within the first 3 days, and the most common choice of specialist was a primary care or sports medicine physician, or a physical therapist. It was also noted that the medical professionals rarely communicated among one another about a dancer patient, nor did they frequently communicate with dance teachers, choreographers, and directors. Interestingly, the dancers surveyed did not think that this communication was vital to their recovery. The dancers in the study did not seem to fully understand their injuries and did not attempt to gain additional information from their health care professionals.

Both dancers and health care professionals reported that additional understanding of anatomy by dancers would be useful.[18]

Professional modern dancers surveyed by Shah and colleagues[4] were queried regarding injury reporting choices, including whether to report to dance company staff and/or to consult medical professionals. Most dancers in this study chose to consult a physician (47%), physical therapist (62%), and chiropractor (34%). Of the 54% of dancers who did not choose to consult a physician, their rationale included not thinking a physician would be helpful (27%), already knowing the diagnosis (19%), not thinking the physician would understand dancers (16%), not having time (9%), not having health insurance (8%), concern of being told to stop dancing for too long (6%), and prior negative experience with a physician (4%). Most of the dancers were noted to have waited between 2 and 7 days before consulting anyone. Dancers in this study were queried about adherence to recommendations. Eighty-seven percent of the male dancers and 78% of the female dancers reported following treatment recommendations, with female dancer compliance remaining consistent and male dancer compliance decreasing for second injury. Reported reasons for not following recommendations included (in descending order) excessive time away from dance, expectation that the injury would improve with time, not wanting staff to know about the injury for concern of not being able to return to class or rehearsal, preference to not take medication, not agreeing with treatment plan, losing a role to another dancer, lack of time for treatments including physical therapy, and a belief that treatments were ineffective.[4]

In a study of collegiate dancers in a university dance program and a performing arts conservatory by Air and colleagues,[28] 36 dancers were prospectively followed and data were collected regarding injury and health care encounters. A high historical (>87%) and current (>55%) injury rate was reported, and most dancers had health insurance and a primary care physician. The dancers expressed a preference for dance teachers as first line in their care (47.5%), followed by physical therapists (30%). Dance teachers, physical therapists, physicians, and dance colleagues all were common (22.5% each) second choices. Dancers who did not choose physicians as one of the top 3 choices were queried as to the rationale for this lack of choice. Although dancers did have confidence in a physician's ability to diagnose and treat, they were not as confident in the doctor's ability to diagnose a dance-related injury and did not expect that the medical doctor would provide a plan but thought the doctor would instead refer them to physical therapy. In making a choice of what type of physician to see, dancers did prefer nonsurgical specialists, including primary care sports medicine physicians and physiatrists, but this was not a major role in selection of a physician. Major factors affecting choice included word of mouth, insurance/cost factors, and prior personal dance experience of the physician. Diagnostic accuracy and feasibility of treatment implementation, along with both inclusion of nonsurgical treatment options and the ability to use and understand dance terminology, were shown to affect the dancers' overall experience. Dancers were also queried about attitudes toward mental health professionals and most (80%) reported they would see a mental health professional if recommended to help cope with a dance-related injury. Of those who would not consider mental health care, reasons included feeling it was unnecessary, lack of time, and cost issues. In the cohort of dancers that sustained injuries over a 6-month period, most who sought treatment were seen by physical therapy or a dance teacher and fewer were seen by a physician, although this did not directly correlate with their preference of treatment provider before injury, possibly influenced by pathways of care with easier access to a nonphysician provider.[28]

Wang and Russell[29] conducted a study of collegiate dancers in 2 different geographic locations within the United States in which the dancers were anonymously surveyed regarding both access to care and level of satisfaction with the care they received. It is noteworthy that a high percentage of these dancers had health insurance coverage (89%), although many dancers (29%) did not seek medical advice from a health care professional for an injury, and 13% did report that cost was a factor in not seeking health care. Other reasons included low injury severity and comfort with self-treatment. Dancers most commonly sought advice from their dance teachers (75%), followed by physicians (59%) and physical therapists (49%). The dancers reported exclusively positive experiences 57% of the time with dance teachers, 45% of the time with physicians, and 67% with physical therapists. Fifty-five percent of the dancers reported negative experiences with the same professionals, with the top 3 reasons being lack of understanding of dancers (70%), providing unhelpful advice (43%), or limited time spent in consultation (33%). For the experiences with health care providers that were reported as positive, the providers were selected by word of mouth or through the provider's institutional affiliation.[29] These findings draw attention to the ongoing barriers between dancers and health care providers, and that more work is needed to improve connection, trust, and quality of care for dancer patients.

AVAILABILITY AND AFFORDABILITY OF HEALTH CARE

Attitudes toward and experience with health care depend on many factors, including geographic region of residence, whether or not a national health care system exists, and access to primary care services and specialty services. In countries with or without a national health care system, various services that may be of use to dancers may not be covered. Third-party payors may shift cost to patients, resulting in increased financial burden of care. In a society where the performing arts may be less recognized or garner less attention than athletics, there may be a disparity between 2 populations that could benefit from similar health care services. In certain countries, such as the United States, workers' compensation may be available at some dance companies, allowing dancers to obtain needed services with less financial burden, including services while performing in geographic locations away from home. Companies with health care professionals on site and who travel with the company can decrease barriers to care. All these factors must be examined in order to build systems of care that optimize availability of services without undue financial burden, whether local or while traveling.

Dancers have their own biases about the health care system, an evolving issue that is highly dependent on geographic location, systems of care, and demographic factors. In order to understand how to help dancers access medical care, an improved understanding of the variety of systems of care is essential. Health care use depends on the respective system in the geographic region where the dancer resides. In a region with universal health care, the perceptions of care may be different from areas with other systems of care. It should also be noted that, even in countries with universal health care, there may be poor access to specialized services. Structure of the local and available health care system can influence dancers' experience and attitudes. Studies of dancer populations within various international regions may shed light on systemic variability in health care delivery. In a study of professional and retired dancers in the Netherlands, where the dancers have access to both universal health care and performing arts specialists, perceptions of the medical profession were examined. Of the preretirement and postretirement dancers completing surveys, financial barriers to receiving health care were not identified, and only a few of the dancers did not have a primary care physician. Overall, the dancers in the study reported a high level of satisfaction with the health care they received. Differences were noted in the older (average age 50 years, range 35–75 years) and younger (average age 21 years, range 9–34 years) dancer groups, including older dancers being more likely to dance while injured, and were more likely to wait before presenting for medical care, and were more comfortable waiting to see whether injury would resolve independently of medical care.[25]

In a study of the demographics and training characteristics of professional modern dancers employed by dance companies in the United States, 18% of the dancers did not have health insurance coverage. Twenty-three percent purchased their own coverage, and 22% had insurance coverage as part of their family's policy, whereas 16% had coverage under workers' compensation. Fifty-four percent of dancers had their employer provide some coverage.[5] This finding shows the financial burden limiting access to care among the high-injury-risk professional modern dance population. Although most employers in the United States are required to provide workers' compensation coverage, it is possible that, because many dancers are part time, freelance, or independent contractors, they are less likely to have access to health care coverage.[5]

Programs delivering on-site health care services to dance companies and schools have gained increasing attention over the past decade, and comprehensive services, including preseason screening, physical therapy, and health care while on tour and backstage, have documented benefit in a large professional modern dance company in the United States, with a reduction in injury rates, lost work days, and workers' compensation claims.[7–9]

In an effort to reduce health care cost in a professional ballet company in the United States, Solomon[11] investigated methods to meet the medical needs of dancers while reducing the financial burden induced by insurance premiums. By contracting health care providers directly by the company to treat dancers on referral by the company physician, providers were paid directly, whereas only major health care expenses had workers' compensation claims. The result was a reduction of expense to the dance company, while concurrently having a positive effect on company morale.[11]

ACCESS TO AND USE OF PRIMARY CARE SERVICES

The value of primary care services is well understood with regard to screening, preventive services, and routine care. Disordered eating and menstrual irregularities occur frequently in dancers and are common in professional dancers and dance students (13.6%–26.5% point prevalence in dance students and 50% lifetime prevalence in professional dancers), and 32% of university-level dancers were found to have menstrual disturbance.[30] Disordered eating and menstrual disturbance can indicate risk for low bone mineral density, although it is unclear whether low bone mineral density is prevalent in female dancers.[31] The presence of relative energy deficiency in sport (RED-S) can predispose dancers to a variety of medical problems, including metabolic rate issues, menstrual dysfunction in women, and immune dysfunction, and can also affect cardiovascular health, along with increasing injury risk and affecting performance.[32]

Routine screening for RED-S in dancers and providing education about energy demands and nutrition requirements can be beneficial.[33] Beyond issues related to energy availability and caloric intake, dancers are at risk for micronutrient deficiency, including iron, calcium, and vitamin D.[34] An editorial authored by physicians and athletes advocated a paradigm shift in women's sport to improve health and performance. It emphasized the need for education in the negative effects of calorie restriction, developing and validating diagnostic tools for RED-S, and ensuring the presence of a referral network for treatment.[35] Routine primary care is an opportunity to identify these issues and provide intervention. Improving awareness among health care providers of the dance aesthetic ideal and risk of disordered eating among dancer patients is a necessary step to reduce the harmful impact of this condition.

To gain insight into the primary care and preventive needs of dancers in the United States, Alimena and colleagues[36] conducted a US study examining the use of routine primary care services by professional and recreational dancers. Thirty-seven dancers presenting to a health screening were queried regarding general medical and orthopedic care and injury history, with questions about primary care visits, mental health, gynecologic care, and nutritional health services. Nutritional assessment included questions regarding vitamin D and calcium supplementation and interest in nutritional counseling, whereas psychological assessment included questions about depression, burnout, fatigue, and sleep deprivation. At the time of the study, more than half (62%) of the dancers had health insurance coverage, although only 54% had seen a physician within the past 2 years and had a dental checkup within the year. Gynecologic services were underused, with only 56% of dancers having seen a gynecologist within the past year, 16.7% never having seen a gynecologist, 30% reporting irregular periods, and more than 16% reporting use of birth control. No statistically significant differences were found with respect to health insurance coverage and frequency of primary care visits, dental examinations, or gynecologic care. Although use of preventive services did not seem to be directly related to insurance coverage status, details regarding the type of coverage (comprehensive vs catastrophic, presence of high deductibles) that have financial impact on policy holders were not analyzed. Many dancers reported a desire for psychological support (29.7%), and also reported high levels of fatigue and sleep deprivation (35.1%). The dancers in the study were found to have high use of ergogenic aids, although few reported supplementation with vitamin D or calcium, and, although most did not report smoking, many (32%) reported a history of binge drinking. Most showed an interest in nutritional counseling (73%).[36] This finding suggests that primary care visits are an opportunity to identify lifestyle risk factors and provide educational resources, including appropriate referrals to other professionals who can support nutritional and psychological needs of their dancer patients.

PROFESSIONAL SOCIETIES AND PUBLIC HEALTH INITIATIVES

There are numerous organizations devoted to collaboration and knowledge exchange among professionals caring for performing artists, ranging from international and national medical professional societies and organizational task forces to local organizations serving dancers in the community. These organizations are driving the future of dancer health and wellness. Programs focused on the optimization of the care of dancers are increasingly found internationally.

Professional societies dedicated to the promotion of dancer health have seen expansion of membership. The International Association for Dance Medicine and Science was formed by 48 members in 1990 as a collaborative effort among dance medicine specialists, dance educators, researchers, and dancers, with the mission to enhance health, well-being, training, and performance of dance by cultivating medical, scientific, and educational excellence. The organization has grown to represent 35 countries and more than 900 members across the globe. Yearly meetings provide opportunity for scientific and clinical presentations, networking, and exchange of ideas. The Web site contains resources for clinicians, educators, and dancers, including pre-pointe readiness and other educational topics, and there is a partnership with Safe in Dance International UK, which offers education and certification to dance educators focused on healthy dance practices.[37] The affiliated publication, the *Journal of Dance Medicine and Science*, is a quarterly international peer-reviewed scientific journal index in Medline.

The Performing Arts Medicine Association was formed in 1988 by physicians involved in the care of musicians and dancers, and grew from a symposium on the Medical Problems of Musicians, which started in 1983. The organization grew beyond physicians to include other health professionals, scientists, performers, and educators. The associated journal, *Medical Problems of Performing Artists*, is the first peer-reviewed journal focused on medical problems affecting dancers, musicians, and actors, and is also the official publication for the Dutch Performing Arts Medicine Association and the Australian Society for Performing Arts Healthcare.

Public health initiatives, including Athletes and the Arts and Dance/USA Task Force on Dancer Health, are instrumental in creating awareness and developing tools by which the dancer population health can improve. The Dance/USA Task Force on Dancer Health focuses on injury and illness prevention. As part of Dance/USA, an organization focusing on engagement through education and programs, advocacy in public policy, research, and preservation of dance legacy through archives, the Task Force consists of volunteer health care professionals who seek to promote the health and safety of professional dancers. Members of the Task Force have collaborated with the American Guild of Musical Artists dancers' union, and work directly with dance companies throughout the United States. Members include physicians, physical therapists, athletic trainers, and chiropractors. Initiatives put forth by the Dance/USA Task Force on Dancer Health include addressing major health issues that affect dancers, including efforts in smoking cessation, addressing disordered eating, promoting nutrition, mental health, and developing a method by which to screen dancers and provide feedback that benefits the individual dancers. Educational information for dancers written by dance medicine specialists is available on the Web site, covering a variety of relevant dancer health topics.[38]

Athletes and the Arts is an initiative based on the premise that athletes and performing artists share many of the same issues, and that performing artists and the sports medicine community benefit mutually from collaboration. Similarities of athletes and performing artists include competitive training environment, high rigor with limited off season, tendency to play/perform through pain, and the ever-present potential for catastrophic injury. Because performing artists tend to be underserved, sports medicine professionals may help bridge the gap by applying principles of sports medicine tailored to the performing artist. Goals of this initiative include incentivizing performing artists to focus on wellness and prevention, educating health care professionals with performing artist patients, and providing a platform via a Web site that allows access to research and educational and clinical resources.[39]

There are multiple medical specialties that are involved in the care of dancers, including orthopedic surgery, internal medicine, family medicine, and physiatry. Physiatry is a specialty suited to serve the needs of dancers because of its team-based, comprehensive approach to care, with a focus on nonsurgical treatment options and also partnering with surgeons to help with return-to-dance rehabilitation. Collaboration with allied health professionals, including physical and occupational therapists, is fundamental to physiatric practice and optimizing dancer health. The

American Academy of Physical Medicine and Rehabilitation has a special-interest community group for performing arts medicine, which was formed to facilitate networking among physiatrist members with clinical interest in the performing arts.[40]

Outside of dance companies with larger budgets that can employ medical staff to provide services for dancers, there has been a grassroots effort on the part of individual health care providers to address the needs of patients in the performing arts. Many clinicians with a passion for dance, often with personal dance experience, offer services on a volunteer basis with the gratification of being able to care for this special population. These clinicians have founded free clinics, provided educational outreach and on-site services, and have made themselves available for dancers to access care in a timely fashion. Although companies with small operating budgets may not be able to provide fee for service for health care professionals, clinicians have many benefits of involvement, including viewing of performances and rehearsals.

HEALTH CARE ADVANCEMENTS AND SYSTEM CHANGE

Health care systems are rapidly changing and there are many forces driving this phenomenon. The growth in technology has been vastly influential in the evolution of health care, including dissemination of health information leading to increased sense of autonomy by patients. Development and widespread use of electronic health records has created the ability of patients to connect with health care providers via secure direct email.[41] This ability can facilitate dancers' connection with their health care providers without taking time away from dance-related activities, allowing clinicians to provide triage and recommend in-person visits if necessary. Furthermore, future growth of telehealth services may benefit dancers who can connect virtually with health care providers when possible, allowing the dancers to maintain a full class and rehearsal schedule.

Technology has resulted in an improved ability to image injuries, which has in turn led to the need for appropriate clinical application to avoid overuse. In particular, musculoskeletal ultrasonography has affected the ability to diagnose both acute and chronic athletic injuries, and to guide interventional procedures that benefit the dancer patient population. Physicians with skills in this technique have additional tools in their armamentarium. There have also been shifts in care initiated through efforts to reduce cost of care, including less one-on-one physician patient care and an increase in team-based care, including nonphysician providers/allied health care. This multilayered approach can result in a system of care with multiple providers offering various services and easier access. If done effectively with clear lines of communication among team members, this may be helpful for dancers looking to various professionals for their health care needs, including educators and health care providers.

The presence of easily accessed information on the Internet allows dancers to find information on symptoms and conditions without seeking services from a health care professional. Physicians often have concerns about the process of self-diagnosis resulting in increased anxiety, excessive concern about conditions, inaccurate diagnosis, and interference with the provider-patient relationship.[42,43] The Internet is a popular source of health information, with variable quality of information. It can be helpful for health care professionals to guide patients to appropriate sources of information.[44] Opportunities for education of dancers in health optimization and preventive care, done by clinical outreach experts, may help mitigate negative outcomes that result from delays in care. Performing arts medicine programs within academic medical institutions, community programs, and programs housed within companies can provide a valuable bridge for facilitating early identification and timely treatment of medical problems. Technological innovations within health and wellness systems, including online systems, telehealth, and mobile device apps, may have the potential to provide injury prevention education and monitoring.[45] Such advances may hold promise in reducing the cost of medical services to performing artists.

SUMMARY

Health care providers with a passion for the performing arts can provide a valuable service and make a difference in the physical, mental, and psychological health of this unique population. Physicians who seek additional training and experience with the clinical care of dancers are well positioned to make an impact on the well-being of dancers, which in turn affects society at large. Understanding dancers' needs and experiences; being able to communicate effectively in their language of dance; willingness to volunteer; and reaching out to schools, training programs, and companies all can help bridge real and perceived gaps in access to care. Furthermore, honing clinical and interventional skills, designing effective treatment plans, and building teams of care providers can benefit local dance communities. Connecting nationally and internationally with similarly interested colleagues allows the sharing of the most current information and ideas with dancer patients. As performing arts medicine continues to grow, health care providers can work together to ensure dancers worldwide have optimal health.

DISCLOSURE

The author has nothing to disclose.

REFERENCES

1. Hincapie CA, Morton EJ, Cassidy JD. Musculoskeletal injuries and pain in dancers: a systematic review. Arch Phys Med Rehabil 2008;89(9):1819–29.
2. Jacobs CL, Hincapié CA, Cassidy JD. Musculoskeletal injuries and pain in dancers: a systematic review update. J Dance Med Sci 2012;16(2):74–84.
3. Shah S. Caring for the dancer: special considerations for the performer and troupe. Curr Sports Med Rep 2008;7(3):128–32.
4. Shah S, Weiss DS, Burchette RJ. Injuries in professional modern dancers: incidence, risk factors, and management. J Dance Med Sci 2012;16(1):17–25.
5. Weiss DS, Shah S, Burchette RJ. A profile of the demographics and training characteristics of professional modern dancers. J Dance Med Sci 2008;12(2):41–6.
6. Garrick JG, Requa RK. Ballet injuries. An analysis of epidemiology and financial outcome. Am J Sports Med 1993;21(4):586–90.
7. Bronner S, Ojofeitimi S, Rose D. Injuries in a modern dance company: effect of comprehensive management on injury incidence and time loss. Am J Sports Med 2003;31(3):365–73.
8. Bronner S, McBride C, Gill A. Musculoskeletal injuries in professional modern dancers: a prospective cohort study of 15 years. J Sports Sci 2018;36(16): 1880–8.
9. Ojofeitimi S, Bronner S. Injuries in a modern dance company effect of comprehensive management on injury incidence and cost. J Dance Med Sci 2011; 15(3):116–22.
10. Gamboa JM, Roberts LA, Maring J, et al. Injury patterns in elite preprofessional ballet dancers and the utility of screening programs to identify risk characteristics. J Orthop Sports Phys Ther 2008;38(3):126–36.

11. Solomon R, Solomon J, Micheli L, et al. The "cost" of injuries in a professional ballet company: a five year study. Med Probl Perform Art 1999;14(4):164–9.

12. Smith PJ, Gerrie BJ, Varner KE, et al. Incidence and prevalence of musculoskeletal injury in ballet: a systematic review. Orthop J Sports Med 2015;3(7). 2325967115592621.

13. Smith TO, Davies L, de Medici A, et al. Prevalence and profile of musculoskeletal injuries in ballet dancers: a systematic review and meta-analysis. Phys Ther Sport 2016;19:50–6.

14. Allen N, Nevill A, Brooks J, et al. Ballet injuries: injury incidence and severity over 1 year. J Orthop Sports Phys Ther 2012;42(9):781–90.

15. Ramkumar PN, Farber J, Arnouk J, et al. Injuries in a professional ballet dance company: a 10-year retrospective study. J Dance Med Sci 2016;20(1):30–7.

16. Liederbach M, Hagins M, Gamboa JM, et al. Assessing and reporting dancer capacities, risk factors, and injuries: recommendations from the IADMS standard measures consensus initiative. J Dance Med Sci 2012;16(4):139–53.

17. Kenny SJ, Palacios-Derflingher L, Whittaker JL, et al. The influence of injury definition on injury burden in preprofessional ballet and contemporary dancers. J Orthop Sports Phys Ther 2018;48(3):185–93.

18. Lai RY, Krasnow D, Thomas M. Communication between medical practitioners and dancers. J Dance Med Sci 2008;12(2):47–53.

19. Vassallo AJ, Pappas E, Stamatakis E, et al. Injury fear, stigma, and reporting in professional dancers. Saf Health Work 2019;10(3):260–4.

20. Krasnow D. Psychology of dealing with the injured dancer. Med Probl Perform Art 1994;9:7–9.

21. Kelman BB. Occupational hazards in female ballet dancers. Advocate for a forgotten population. AAOHN J 2000;48(9):430–4.

22. Hamilton LH, Hamilton WG, Meltzer JD, et al. Personality, stress, and injuries in professional ballet dancers. Am J Sports Med 1989;17(2):263–7.

23. Anderson R, Hanrahan SJ. Dancing in pain: pain appraisal and coping in dancers. J Dance Med Sci 2008;12(1):9–16.

24. Wainwright SP, Williams C, Turner BS. Fractured identities: injury and the balletic body. Health (London) 2005;9(1):49–66.

25. Air M. Health care seeking behavior and perceptions of the medical profession among pre- and post-retirement age Dutch dancers. J Dance Med Sci 2009; 13(2):42–50.

26. Nordin-Bates SM, Walker IJ, Baker J, et al. Injury, imagery, and self-esteem in dance healthy minds in injured bodies? J Dance Med Sci 2011;15(2):76–85.

27. Laws H. Fit to dance 2. Report of the second national inquiry into dancers' health and injury in the UK. Birmingham: Dance UK; 2005.

28. Air ME, Grierson MJ, Davenport KL, et al. Dissecting the doctor-dancer relationship: health care decision making among American collegiate dancers. PM R 2014;6(3):241–9.

29. Wang TJ, Russell JA. A tenuous pas de deux: examining university dancers' access to and satisfaction with healthcare delivery. Med Probl Perform Art 2018; 33(2):111–7.

30. Hincapie CA, Cassidy JD. Disordered eating, menstrual disturbances, and low bone mineral density in dancers: a systematic review. Arch Phys Med Rehabil 2010;91(11):1777–89.e1.

31. Amorim T, Wyon M, Maia J, et al. Prevalence of low bone mineral density in female dancers. Sports Med 2015;45(2):257–68.

32. Mountjoy M, Sundgot-Borgen JK, Burke LM, et al. IOC consensus statement on relative energy deficiency in sport (RED-S): 2018 update. Br J Sports Med 2018;52(11):687–97.
33. Civil R, Lamb A, Loosmore D, et al. Assessment of dietary intake, energy status, and factors associated with red-s in vocational female ballet students. Front Nutr 2018;5:136.
34. Sousa M, Carvalho P, Moreira P, et al. Nutrition and nutritional issues for dancers. Med Probl Perform Art 2013;28(3):119–23.
35. Ackerman KE, Stellingwerff T, Elliott-Sale KJ, et al. REDS (Relative Energy Deficiency in Sport): time for a revolution in sports culture and systems to improve athlete health and performance. Br J Sports Med 2020;54(7):369–70.
36. Alimena S, Air ME, Gribbin C, et al. Utilization of routine primary care services among dancers. J Dance Med Sci 2016;20(3):95–102.
37. International association for dance medicine & science. Available at: https://www.iadms.org/. Accessed April 24, 2020.
38. Dance/USA task force on dancer health. Available at: https://www.danceusa.org/dancerhealth. Accessed April 24, 2020.
39. Athletes and the arts. Available at: http://athletesandthearts.com/. Accessed April, 2020.
40. American Academy of physical medicine & rehabilitation: active member communities. Available at: https://www.aapmr.org/about-aapm-r/membership/member-communities/all-member-communities#PerformingArts. Accessed April, 2020.
41. Dendere R, Slade C, Burton-Jones A, et al. Patient portals facilitating engagement with inpatient electronic medical records: a systematic review. J Med Internet Res 2019;21(4):e12779.
42. Jutel A. "Dr. Google" and his predecessors. Diagnosis (Berl) 2017;4(2):87–91.
43. White RW, Horvitz E. Experiences with web search on medical concerns and self diagnosis. AMIA Annu Symp Proc 2009;2009:696–700.
44. Morahan-Martin JM. How internet users find, evaluate, and use online health information: a cross-cultural review. Cyberpsychol Behav 2004;7(5):497–510.
45. Dorsey ER, Topol EJ. State of telehealth. N Engl J Med 2016;375(14):1400.

A Call for Active Resilience Training in Dance

David M. Popoli, MD[a,b,c,d],*

KEYWORDS

- Resilience • Emotional resilience • Cognitive resilience • Spiritual resilience
- Physical resilience • Psychological resilience • Potentially adverse event
- Transitions

KEY POINTS

- Dancers experience significant physical and psychological demands that can be detrimental to health and performance.
- Potentially adverse events often occur at key career inflection points including amateur to preprofessional, preprofessional to professional, and professional to retirement.
- Dancers can build their physical and psychological resilience to reduce negative impacts.
- The Active Resilience Training in Dance curriculum can provide dancers with efficient, timely, and career-specific instruction.

INTRODUCTION AND BACKGROUND

Merriam Webster defines resilience as "the capability of a strained body to recover its size and shape after deformation caused especially by compressive stress" or alternatively, "an ability to recover from or adjust easily to misfortune or change."[1] The latter definition is likely the more familiar to most of us; this is what many call "grit," "mental toughness," or "resolve." The first definition, however, is equally important, although it requires some translation out of its physics scope; in a broader context, it applies to the concept of physical recovery. When considered together, the 2 definitions suggest that resilience has essential psychological and physical components.

Resilience has an impact on an individual's response to potentially adverse events, and physical injury,[2] emotional stress,[3,4] altered sleep,[5] inadequate nutrition,[6] and

[a] Department of Orthopedics, Wake Forest Baptist Health, 1 Medical Center Boulevard, 8th Floor Janeway Tower, Winston Salem, NC 27157, USA; [b] Department of Pediatrics, Wake Forest Baptist Health, 1 Medical Center Boulevard, 8th Floor Janeway Tower, Winston Salem, NC 27157, USA; [c] Division of PM&R, Wake Forest Baptist Health, 1 Medical Center Boulevard, 8th Floor Janeway Tower, Winston Salem, NC 27157, USA; [d] Division of Sports Medicine, Wake Forest Baptist Health, 1 Medical Center Boulevard, 8th Floor Janeway Tower, Winston Salem, NC 27157, USA
* Division of Sports Medicine, Wake Forest Baptist Health, 1 Medical Center Boulevard, 8th Floor Janeway Tower, Winston Salem, NC 27157.
E-mail address: dpopoli@wakehealth.edu

Phys Med Rehabil Clin N Am 32 (2021) 35–49
https://doi.org/10.1016/j.pmr.2020.09.009
1047-9651/21/© 2020 Elsevier Inc. All rights reserved.

performance failure[7] have been proposed as surrogate markers of declining resilience. Popular media abounds with stories of burnout, generational changes in stress and anxiety levels, and declining satisfaction in work-life balance. In medicine, the topic has piqued the interest of the American Medical Association, American College of Surgeons, Association of American Medical Colleges, and The Council of Faculty and Academic Societies. In recent work published in the Mayo Clinic Proceedings, one researcher found that 54.4% of physicians surveyed in 2014 reported at least 1 symptom of burnout, an increase from 45.5% in 2011. 46.9% reported emotional exhaustion, 39.8% screened positive for depression, and only 10.6% reported having enough personal/family time.[8] Physicians cited factors including excessive work hours, complex decision-making, difficulty separating personal and professional lives, and depersonalization as major challenges to their resilience.[9] Consequently, the field of medicine has seen a steep rise in wellness initiatives, peer-support programs, and formal resilience seminars designed to deflect negative impacts.

Dancers, like physicians, are asked to meld career and personhood, and they face similar challenges: irregular work hours, emotionally taxing work, and the pressures of perfectionism. Also like physicians, they report increased levels of burnout and depression as manifestations of strained psychological resilience. Unlike medical professionals, however, elite dancers also assume the bodily risks of an athletic career, including repetitive load and demanding mechanics, that can challenge physical resilience. They, too, would benefit from resilience training programs like those offered to medical professionals, albeit with dance-specific considerations.

This article provides an overview of some of the physical and psychological challenges that dancers face at key inflection points in their careers and considers a response triad of actions, belief, and behaviors (**Fig. 1**) to build and maintain the core domains of resilience (**Fig. 2**). The composite program is called Active Resilience Training in Dance (ART).

KEY INFLECTION POINTS THAT CHALLENGE DANCER RESILIENCE

Some dance companies have taken initial steps to address resilience in their dancers, often in the form of global "wellness" programs. At present, however, this is generally limited to basic discussion. Resilience training efforts are not generally time-specific or consistent. Consequently, resilience gaps may develop and can result in preventable cases of burnout or diminished performance quality at the following inflection points:

Amateur/Preprofessional: Volume and Vigor

When new to the preprofessional rank, many dancers struggle with the volume of choreography and the increased physical demands on their bodies. Stress can be compounded by feelings of insecurity due to a heightened awareness of similarly gifted colleagues. Escalating expectations paired with a desire to remain "the best" can shake self-esteem and generate unhealthy competition. Resilience training at this stage would help mitigate overload and promote comradery.

Preprofessional/Professional: Locus and Focus

The transition to professional dance poses a significant challenge. Time demands dramatically increase, and many dancers experience role assignments as being arbitrary or solely based on seniority. This can generate feelings of lost autonomy, disconnection from the artform, or a sacrifice of artistic purity.[10] In addition, the transition from preprofessional to professional shifts the focus from the group to the individual. A dancer secures his or her roles not via by company cohesion but by outstanding

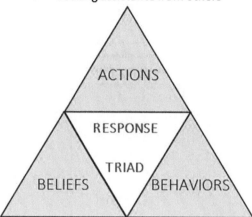

Examples:
- ➤ Goal-setting
- ➤ Analysis of failure
- ➤ Seeking assistance from others

Examples:
- ➤ Self-worth
- ➤ Core values
- ➤ Situational mutability

Examples:
- ➤ Learning personal and group strength/weaknesses
- ➤ Confronting challenges
- ➤ Recognizing and addressing own emotions and those of others

Fig. 1. Resilience-building triad.

individual performance. To an individual accustomed to success or failure that is largely determined by group effort, shifting to a more singular focus can be an adjustment. Resilience training at this stage would help dancers cultivate perspective and maintain core values.

Professional/Retirement: Reality and Reinvention

For most dancers, retirement is the most anxiety-provoking transition. They are now "ex-athletes," both literally and symbolically. They must address the physical toll that dance may have exacted on their bodies and confront the emotional challenge of a career change. They are no longer the purveyors of their art but rather ambassadors. Dancers may struggle with finding fulfilling outlets for their skill set or may be intimidated by the thought of developing a new one. Resilience training at this stage would help reinforce self-worth and encourage self-discovery.

ASSESSMENT OF RESILIENCE

Although dancers' work with technique instructors or artistic directors may reveal their personality and "grit," there is no objective assessment of resilience. Without any knowledge of "at-risk" dancers or data trends, a dance company, therefore, has a limited ability to intervene with workshops or counseling. The opportunity, therefore, is twofold. First, assessment of resilience at strategic inflection points could help a

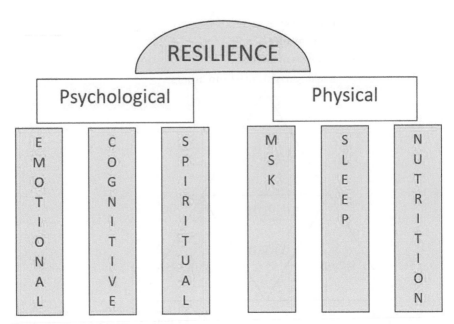

Fig. 2. Resilience domains.

conservatory or company understand common vulnerabilities and identify dancers who would benefit from assistance. Second, the data collected could, in turn, be used to hone a curriculum designed to promote and support resilience during these stressful transitions.

In an effort to provide a measure of global resilience (trait) and likely response strategies to potentially adverse events (state), dancers would be asked to complete 2 brief questionnaires, the Brief Resilience Scale (BRS)[11] and the Brief Resilience Coping Scale (BRCS).[12] Initially, these metrics would serve as a "baseline" value for an individual at each key career inflection discussed previously. Dancers would then be asked to repeat the questionnaires at 2 other fixed time points (1 month and 6 months after the completion of the resilience curriculum). All data collection would be electronic via Survey Monkey or RedCap, and identifiable data would be available only to teaching faculty for the purposes of academic support. De-identified data would be stored electronically for analysis and research.

The Brief Resilience Scale

The BRS (**Table 1**)[11] was developed in 2008 by researchers in the Department of Psychology at the University of New Mexico. Their aim was to create a tool that directly measured resilience, defined in their study as the "ability to bounce or spring back-...from stress." Their team argued that previous tools to measure resilience focused too heavily on "factors and resources that make [resilience] possible."[11] They wanted a more direct measure. Their validation study, published in the *International Journal of Behavioral Medicine*, demonstrates that a 6-question assessment (shown later in this article) takes an accurate measure of "true" resilience and controls for other factors such as social support, optimism, and substance use/abuse.

To each of the statements listed, the subject replies on a 1 to 5 Likert Scale (strongly disagree, disagree, neutral, agree, strongly agree), and responses are

Items	Sample 1	Sample 2	Sample 3	Sample 4
Table 1 **The brief resilience scale: items and factor lodgings**				
1. I tend to bounce back quickly after hard times	.77	.79	.70	.89
2. I have a hard time making it through stressful events (R)	.73	.78	.68	.91
3. It does not take me long to recover from a stressful event	.78	.78	.71	.71
4. It is hard for me to snap back when something bad happens (R)	.85	.90	.70	.85
5. I usually come through difficult times with little trouble	.69	.69	.71	.68
6. I tend to take a long time to get over setbacks in my life (R)	.84	.81	.67	.68

Note. Sample 1 = 128 undergraduate students; Sample 2 = 64 undergraduate students; Sample 3 = 112 cardiac rehabilitation patients; Sample 4 = 50 women with fibromyalgia or healthy controls. R = reverse coded items.

From Smith BW, Dalen J, Wiggins K, et al. The brief resilience scale: assessing the ability to bounce back. Int J Behav Med. 2008;15: 194–200; with permission.

summed (reverse coded for questions 2, 4, and 6) and divided by 6 to obtain a mean. The maximum ("most resilient") score is a 5. In several additional validation studies conducted after the introduction of the BRS, the mean varies between approximately 2.8 and 3.0. This tool, then, would be used in the ART program as a direct measure of the trait of resilience and would be expected to remain constant.

The Brief Resilience Coping Scale

The BRCS (**Table 2**)[12] was developed at Vanderbilt University in an effort to measure "the patterns of resilience, more specifically the situational pattern, which corresponds to resilient coping patterns...including tenacity, optimism, creativity, an aggressive approach to problem solving, and commitment to positive growth from difficult situations."[13] Unlike the BRS, it is intended to identify behaviors or strategies that enhance resilience and would be expected to change with training.

To each of the statements listed previously, the subject replies on a 1 to 5 Likert scale with the instructions "Consider how well the following statements describe your behavior and actions on a scale from 1 to 5, where 1 means the statement does not describe you at all and 5 means it describes you very well."[12] Numerical values are then summed. The maximum (most resilient coping pattern) score is a 20. According to the original investigators, those with a score from 0 to 13 were "at risk," scores from 14 to 17 were considered "moderately resilient," and scores greater than 17 were "highly resilient."[12] Researchers have also found that BRCS scores respond to cognitive-behavioral interventions,[12–14] and therefore this scale will be helpful to determine the impact of the curriculum intervention.

If a dancer expresses concern about his or her score on the BRS/BRCS, the ART in Dance program could assist in arranging supplemental meetings with a sports psychologist or Wellness Center, depending on the circumstances. All dancers would be encouraged to view their scores not as a predictor of success or failure but rather as an opportunity for personal reflection and development.

Table 2
BRCS item wording, means, standard deviations, item-total correlations, and Cronbach's Alpha if item is deleted

Item Wording	Mean		SD		Corrected Item— Total Correlation		Alpha If Item Deleted	
	S1	S2	S1	S2	S1	S2	S1	S2
I look for creative ways to alter difficult situations.	4.15	3.73	0.91	1.10	0.45	0.49	0.70	0.61
Regardless of what happens to me. I believe I can control my reaction to it.	3.57	3.50	0.93	1.02	0.46	0.40	0.70	0.66
I believe I can grow in positive ways by dealing with difficult situations.	4.14	3.88	0.88	0.84	0.55	0.50	0.65	0.61
I actively look for ways to replace the losses 1 encounter in life.	3.69	3.45	1.01	1.08	0.61	0.49	0.61	0.60

Abbreviations: BRCS, Brief Resilience Coping Scale; SI, Sample I; S2, Sample 2.
From Sinclair VG, Wallston KA. The development and psychometric evaluation of the brief resilient coping scale. Assessment. 2004;11(1):94-101; with permission.

Physical Resilience

Although there is not a gold standard measure of physical resilience, longitudinal tracking of injury rates and mean recovery times could serve as surrogate markers. Injury, in this setting, would be defined as any condition that prevented a dancer from participating fully in normally scheduled dance activities for at least 24 hours from the time of the inciting event.[15] This definition has been proposed by Allen and colleagues[15] and is routinely used in dance medicine literature, expressed in the common sports medicine format of injuries per athlete hour of exposure. Dancers' rate of injury before the ART in Dance curriculum could be interpreted as their collective resistance to an adverse physical stress, and injury rates could be tracked over time to determine if physical resilience training could be part of a solution.

In addition to injury rate, the percentage of dancers who return to sport after injury and their mean recovery time would also be tracked. These metrics represent a dancer's ability to respond to, and recover from, the adverse physical stress. Return to sport would be reported as a percentage of individuals who return to dance without restriction. Mean recovery time would be measured in days.

ACTIVE RESILIENCE TRAINING IN DANCE CURRICULUM OVERVIEW
Design Concept

The ART in Dance program will comprise four 90-minute seminars derived, in part, from the Penn Resilience Program,[16] and deployed at 3 time points selected for specific challenges to resilience. These times are often associated with heightened anxiety, self-doubt, and fear of the unknown, therefore assessing for and promoting resilience in sync with periods of risk represents an opportunity to intervene proactively. Initially, traveling trainers would lead the curriculum; however, future cycles could be taught in-house.

ART in Dance curriculum is designed to move longitudinally with the learner and to coincide with 3 key career inflection points:

- Amateur to Preprofessional
- Preprofessional to Professional
- Professional to Retirement

The goal of the ART in Dance curriculum is to provide progressive instruction. Each stage of learning would build on the last and include both didactic and experiential components. Didactics would be delivered by content experts from both within and outside of dance. Experiential learning would focus on actions, beliefs, and behaviors that foster resilience and could include collaboration with resilience leaders from the fields of medicine, business, or adult learning. Ultimately, the ART in Dance program would help ensure that the next generation of dancers were prepared for career challenges and could give them a performance advantage.

Proposed Teaching Tool

The Penn Resilience Program (PRP)[16] was developed by Drs. Seligman, Reivich, and Gillham to address and improve the psychological response to adversity. This program has 5 modules and has generally been delivered in twelve 90-minute sessions or eighteen to twenty-four 60-minute sessions over the span of several months. Modules include the following:

1. *Emotional fitness*: how to amplify positive emotions and recognize when negative ones are out of proportion to the threat being faced.
2. *Family fitness*: focuses on relationship skills including fostering trust, constructively managing conflict, and creating shared meaning.
3. *Social fitness*: teaches empathy and asks participants to practice identifying emotions in others with the goal of developing "emotional intelligence."
4. *Spiritual fitness*: teaches self-awareness, self-regulation, self-motivation, and social awareness. Spiritual, in this training course, "refers not to religion but to belonging to and serving something larger than self."
5. *Posttraumatic growth*: understanding the response to trauma, reducing anxiety through techniques for controlling intrusive thoughts, engaging in constructive self-disclosure, and "creating a narrative in which the trauma is seen as a fork in the road that enhances life."

The program has been tested in diverse settings ranging from middle school adolescents in inner cities to the "Comprehensive Solider Fitness" initiative for the US military. A meta-analysis from 2009 that combined the results of 17 studies of the Penn Resilience Program (PRP) studies with a total 2489 participants demonstrated that the program had a probability of superiority (PS) score ranging from 0.33 to 0.66 (CI 0.11–0.33).[17] PS score reflects the probability that a randomly selected PRP participant would have a favorable outcome after a potentially adverse event as compared with a randomly selected control participant. A PS score of 0.50, therefore, indicates that there is 50% chance that a randomly selected PRP participant has a better score than a randomly selected control participant (ie, no intervention effect).

Adaptation of the Penn Resilience Program as a Foundation for Active Resilience Training in Dance

The PRP would be scaled down for the ART in Dance program; several of the major concepts from the PRP would be combined under the umbrella term *psychological resilience* (see **Fig. 1**) and discussed as the following subgroups:

1. *Emotional Resilience*: the ability to identify and address negative emotions, modulate response to stress, and recognize emotional "choke points" that inhibit personal and professional growth.
2. *Cognitive Resilience*: the ability to maintain concentration/focus, identify alternative pathways to address complex problems, and maintain objectivity after failure.
3. *Spiritual Resilience*: the ability to maintain a sense of self-worth, act purposefully in accordance with a set of values, and derive meaning from potentially adverse events.

Given the profession of the intended audience, the ART in Dance program would add a major category, *physical resilience*, to account for the physical demands placed on this unique group of athletes and to promote long-term investment in whole-body wellness. Training and discussion would include the following:

- *Musculoskeletal Health*: overview of acute and overuse injury involving muscle, bone, and joint and discussion/implementation of cross-training concepts.
- *Nutrition*: discussion of general nutrition concepts, fueling requirements, and nutritional influences on injury risk and performance.
- *Sleep*: discussion of sleep schedules and exploration of sleep's impact on performance and injury risk.

Whereas the PRP runs for several months and up to 24 sessions, the ART in Dance program would be condensed into four, 90-minute mini-seminars comprising the 2 primary domains and their associated subcategories listed previously.

PSYCHOLOGICAL RESILIENCE
Lesson 1: Emotional Resilience

Didactic instruction for this module would draw from the principles of Rational Emotive Behavior Therapy and Cognitive Therapy. Dancers would learn the some of the foundations of these therapies, including the impact of distorted perceptions and the way in which irrational beliefs can lead to the creation of negative emotions in response to a potentially adverse event. Specifically, dancers would be asked to learn the ABC portion of the ABCDE Model, initially proposed by Albert Ellis in 1957 and refined over the past 60+ years (**Fig. 3**).[18]

Once familiar with the model, dancers would apply it to real-life scenarios specific to the key career inflection point at which the curriculum was delivered. Ideally, these would be drawn from recent experiences and would therefore allow for a high degree of personalization and practical utility. During this session, each dancer would initially work through the ABC portion of the ABCDE model using a Situational Awareness Worksheet (**Table 3**).[19]

For example, a dancer might report a poor performance at a recent audition as an activating event (A). He or she would then write down the consequence or consequences (C) of that event. Perhaps he or she felt depressed for several days afterward, had a conflict with a family member, or consumed an abnormal amount of alcohol. That individual would then reflect back on the belief (B) that led to the consequence; for example, feeling that every audition must be perfect in order to get a job or that a poor performance makes him or her worthless.

At this point, the exercise would turn to small-group work to discuss the beliefs that led to the undesirable consequence. This element of the curriculum is essential. Those enrolled would practice self-reflection and constructive coaching, making resilience-building not only a personal but also a group experience. This exercise would encourage dancers to construct supportive social networks and would emphasize

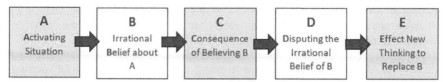

Fig. 3. ABCDE model. (*Data from* Centre for Clinical Interventions. Module 6: Perfectionism in Perspective. Available at: https://www.cci.health.wa.gov.au/~/media/CCI/Consumer% 20Modules/Perfectionism%20in%20Perspective/Perfectionism%20in%20Perspective%20-% 2006%20-%20Challenging%20my%20perfectionistic%20thinking.pdf. Accessed September 8, 2020.)

effective communication strategies and collaboration rather than harsh criticism or competition.

Between this session and the next, participants would be asked to identify, engage in, and record a challenging event using the ABC model. This would allow each dancer to explore a triad of *actions, beliefs, and behaviors* to enhance emotional resilience.

- Actions: Analysis of failure, naming and examining emotional response.
- Beliefs: Introspection, linkage of perception and interpretation of an event.
- Behaviors: Confronting a challenge, productive criticism.

Lesson 2: Cognitive Resilience

Building on the foundation of emotional resilience, the next structural element of the ART in Dance curriculum would be cognitive resilience. This portion would begin with a deeper analysis of the DE components of the ABCDE model. Didactics would focus on the process of disputing unfounded beliefs (D) through evidentiary review

Table 3
Situational analysis worksheet

Activating Situation	*Beliefs*
What happened?	Think about self-statements that link A to C.
• Actual event?	What did you tell yourself?
• Reliving a memory?	Underline the most distressing belief.
I had a Bad audition	Rate (0–10) how strongly you hold this belief.
Consequences	*I am not as good as the other dancers.*
• Write down words that describe	*I do not learn choreography as fast as everyone else.*
how you felt after this situation.	*I am not going to make it to the next level. 9/10*
Depressed 8/10	*Unhelpful Thinking Styles*
Worthless	Note any unhelpful thinking styles that you may
Scared Upset Stomach	have used (eg, catastrophizing, "musting,"
Disappointed	black/white thinking, magnification,
• Underline the word most strongly	minimization, labeling)
associated with the situation.	*Catastrophizing*
• Rate the intensity of this feeling	*Maximization*
from 0 (least intense) to 10	*Black/white thinking*
(most intense)	
• List any physical symptoms you	
experienced during this situation	
(ie, heart racing, headache)	

Data from Strecher VJ. On Purpose: Lessons in Life and Health from the Frog, Dung Beetle, and Julia. Ann Arbor, MI: Dung Beetle Press; 2013.

and then reframing the activating event in a neutral or positive way to effect change (E). The overarching theme would be the use of facts to prevent automatic, emotion-based action or response.

Next, participants would be asked to get out their homework from the previous session (the ABC reflection on a recent event) and work through the DE components of the Resolution Worksheet (**Table 4**).[19] Initially, this would be an individual exercise, however, participants would then be asked to rejoin their respective groups from the previous session to discuss their findings and solicit feedback from others.

In the group setting, dancers would be tasked with identifying coping strategies to mitigate unhelpful thinking and to create a stepwise path to implement change. For example, a group might discuss how mindfulness techniques such as breathing exercises or muscle relaxation techniques could counteract a tendency to become stuck in compulsive thinking. They might also suggest that breaking a desired outcome into small, progressive goals could decrease anxiety and assist in planning.

Table 4
Resolution worksheet

Discovery
  Write down the most distressing belief. What factual evidence is there *for* and *against* this belief?
Most Distressing Belief:
  I am not going to make it to the next level

Factual Evidence For This Belief:	Factual Evidence Against This Belief:
I performed poorly at this audition.	*I usually audition well.*
I have not had lead roles recently.	*I have had many leads in the past.*
I have an ankle injury.	*I have learned a lot in physical therapy.*

Dispute: consider the following questions:	• What positives about myself or this situation am I ignoring due to a negative mindset?
• If I were not feeling emotionally charged, how would I view this situation?	• How might someone else view this situation?
• What are alternative ways of viewing this event?	• How productive is my current mindset in terms of achieving my goals?
• What is the most realistic outcome of this situation?	• What could I tell myself right now to help?

Having a bad audition does not make me a bad dancer.
Everyone has an off-day every once in a while.
If I don't get cast in this show, I will be able to focus more on the other show I'm in.
Being injured has actually taught me a lot about injury prevention and the way I dance.
Telling myself I will fail makes me feel worse and decreases my confidence.

Effect Positive Change
After looking at the factual evidence for and against your most distressing thought, and having considered the reframing questions listed previously, write a new balanced/helpful thought.
Having a bad audition is challenging, particularly while also dealing with an injury, but it will give me opportunities to learn more about myself as a dancer and can help in the future.

Rerate the underlined emotion	Rerate how strongly you hold your belief
from C 5/10	from B 4/10

Data from Centre for Clinical Interventions. Module 6: Perfectionism in Perspective. Available at: https://www.cci.health.wa.gov.au/~/media/CCI/Consumer%20Modules/Perfectionism%20in%20Perspective/Perfectionism%20in%20Perspective%20-%2006%20-%20Challenging%20my%20perfectionistic%20thinking.pdf. Accessed September 8, 2020.

To consolidate learning from this session, participants would analyze a recent setback with the full ABCDE model and then propose a stepwise approach to enacting change. This would include a list of prioritized goals and then a time-specific breakdown of the components necessary to achieve that goal. The *actions, beliefs, and behaviors* covered by the cognitive resilience session would therefore include the following:

- Actions: Using factual evidence to dispute distorted perceptions, creating a roadmap to change.
- Beliefs: Self-empowerment to enact change, internal locus of control.
- Behaviors: Reframing setbacks, generating positive outlook.

Lesson 3: Spiritual Resilience

In the prior emotional and cognitive resilience sessions, participants learned how to use guided introspection (following the ABCDE Model and mindfulness techniques) to create a neutral psychological space in which to examine a potentially adverse event. These skills are important but are not geared toward carry-over. In an effort to promote the long-term utility of the ART in Dance curriculum, the spiritual resilience session would now ask dancers to home in on *why* they experience certain emotions and tend to follow a patterned response. By examining their motivations and identifying their guiding principles, students would create a roadmap of important personal "checkpoints" to consider when facing challenges. This would ensure that any plans put in place were consistent with their core beliefs.

Didactic instruction for this module would be based on the work of Victor Strecher, PhD.[20] As a large group, dancers would produce a list of virtues. This could include words such as creativity, responsibility, community-focused, or enthusiastic. Once the list reaches 20 items, or until the group feels the list is sufficiently diverse and representative of those attending the session, each dancer would then be asked to select between 3 and 5 words that speak of his or her core values and write down why. Next, participants would craft a 1-sentence "self-memoir." How would he or she like to be remembered as a dancer and a person? Strecher[20] describes this as "consider what you'd like to see written on your headstone...what would you want people to read about you?" At this point, dancers would break into small groups (no >6) to discuss the activity. What has each learned? What motivates them, and how do they want to be perceived by others? While still in their small groups, dancers would now be asked to create their purpose statement: an internal philosophy based on their core values and desired persona. These statements would be shared within the small group with adequate time allotted for reflection and discussion.

With purpose statements in hand, dancers would reconvene as a large group, and discussion would shift to an exploration of techniques to help synchronize purpose and action. This section would be multi-modal and could include instruction in mindfulness practices such as controlled breathing or guided imagery to assist dancers in gaining insight. It would also present 2 tools, which would be integrated into assignments after the conclusion of the spiritual resilience session.

The first of these, the Wandering Map, would serve as a verification of the dancer's purpose statement. Sometime before the next session, ART in Dance participants would be asked to start with a blank piece of paper and then quickly fill the page with ideas, names, sketches, short phrases, pictures, song lyrics, etc. that have been important in their lives. Next, they would find connections or themes; some might be obvious (family members) but others less so (love of puzzles, perhaps). At this point, the dancer would compare his or her purpose statement to the Wandering Map to confirm overlap and/or identify bias.

Next, dancers would be asked to check for action/purpose alignment in current daily activities using the Action-Purpose Alignment Tool (**Fig. 4**).[21] For example, a dancer might identify her purpose as "To bring joy to myself and others by sharing artistic expression." Using this as a foundational "checkpoint," she could then examine discreet actions to determine if they aligned with her stated purpose or not. Perhaps she spent 60 hours in rehearsal that week: although this would partially align with artistic expression, it may not bring her joy.

Although this process analysis might initially be awkward, with time and repetition, it would facilitate integration of new behaviors.[21] One group of researchers found that those who demonstrated high levels of adherence to self-transcending guiding principles (empathy, compassion, contribution) were more likely to have achieved their goals at 2 years and to report greater scores of well-being than those who aspired to self-enhancing ones (money, power, status).[22] Actions, beliefs, and behaviors reinforced during the spiritual resilience session would include the following:

- Actions: Thoughtful self-discovery, identifying motivating forces.
- Beliefs: Self-worth, personal vision and mission.
- Behaviors: Grounding actions in core beliefs, filtering events through guiding principles to achieve happiness and success.

Lesson 4: Physical Resilience

This arm of the ART in Dance curriculum would be a review of concepts and practices intended to enhance physical resilience. Although many of the participants would be familiar with these topics, the emphasis would be on integrating actions into daily routine rather than didactic instruction alone.

Musculoskeletal and bone health

The ART in Dance curriculum assumes most dancers will have a basic understanding of musculoskeletal overuse and the concept of cross-training. Didactic instruction for physical resilience, therefore, would not include a review of anatomy or make broad universal statements about the benefits of muscle symmetry or flexibility. Instead, this session would examine some of the most common dance injuries in detail, discuss

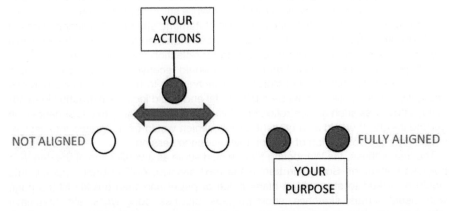

Fig. 4. Action-purpose alignment model. (*Data from* Strecher VJ. On Purpose: Lessons in Life and Health from the Frog, Dung Beetle, and Julia. Ann Arbor, MI: Dung Beetle Press; 2013.)

why overuse and training errors contribute to their occurrence, and identify *how* cross-training mitigates the effect. This would frame cross-training not as an addition to a dancer's already-busy schedule but rather as a constant modifiable risk factor for injury. As such, dancers would be introduced to the concept of "dance breaks": brief (15–30-minute) daily doses of physical activity that break up blocks of dance and encourage the use of other muscle groups. Potential options that have some supporting literature include martial arts,[23] Pilates,[24] and yoga.[24] ART in Dance participants would be asked to engage in 2 to 3 minutes of each of these activities during the session and then reflect on the movements.

Nutrition

This portion of the physical resilience curriculum would present nutrition as a preparatory practice to optimize performance. Participants would learn about fueling principles including energy availability and personalization. There would be no discussion of specific diets, supplements, calorie-counting techniques, or nutrition apps. Facilitators would ask participants to write down their current attitude about food (eg, reward, fuel, enemy) and filter it through the ABCDE Model to search for distorted perceptions and to reframe if appropriate. Dancers would then be asked to apply the Action-Purpose Alignment Tool to their current nutrition habits to provide perspective on possible improvements.

Sleep

Sleep would be presented as a vital component of both physical and psychological resilience. Discussion would center around concepts explored in the work of Fietze and colleagues,[25] who demonstrated that not only did dancers sleep fewer hours leading up to a performance, but that they also experienced impaired sleep quality. Their studies showed that these changes contributed significantly to increased injury and burnout rates.[25] Similar to the way in which nutrition was discussed, sleep would be framed in terms of performance optimization and risk modification. Facilitators would not discuss an "optimal" number of sleep hours; dancers would be asked to review their current sleep hygiene in terms of consistency and sufficiency to achieve performance goals. Dancers may choose to deploy the Action-Purpose Alignment Tool for objective confirmation.

Taken in sum, actions, beliefs, and behaviors addressed during the physical resilience session would include the following:

- Actions: Integrating consistent cross-training, aligning nutrition and sleep habits with career goals.
- Beliefs: Whole-body preparation for elite physical activity, informed habits instead of trends.
- Behaviors: Challenging engrained choices for calories and sleep hours, seeking fun in nondance activities.

ANALYSIS

Pre- and post-curricular BRS and BCRS scores would be collected to determine the effect size at each intervention point. In addition, BRS/BCRS scores would be tracked longitudinally to ascertain the potential benefit of repeat exposure to the ART curriculum. There may be an opportunity to analyze resilience data against other indices, such as the Athlete Burnout Inventory, Beck Depression Inventory, or the Short Form 12 (SF-12) Health Survey. In addition to BRS and BCRS scores, injury data, including rates and mean recovery times, would be collected longitudinally. Results of all analyses would be collated, analyzed for trends, and used not only to improve the program in which it was deployed but also shared with the Dance Medicine community via scientific presentation or submitted to a peer-reviewed journal for publication.

SUMMARY

Over the course of their careers, dancers face several key inflection points. These transitions often create physical and psychological strain that can hamper performance and increase the risk of injury. The ART in Dance curriculum seeks to measure baseline resilience and coping strategies, provide curriculum to address key pillars of psychological and physical resilience, and track metrics over time to hone the program. ART in Dance places an emphasis on a triad of attitudes, beliefs, and behaviors that can be integrated into daily life so that instruction becomes part of a dancer's routine. Potential benefits include the following:

For the dancer: Decreased injury risk, increased situational control, enhanced performance.

For the dance company: Decreased role substitutions, decreased cost, increased recruiting appeal.

CLINICS CARE POINTS

- Check dancer resilience with an evidence-based tool such as the BRS or BCRS.
- Treat resilience as a risk-factor for injury.

DISCLOSURE

The author has no financial or commercial disclosures.

REFERENCES

1. "Resilience." The Merriam-Webster.com Dictionary, Merriam-Webster Inc.. Available at: https://www.merriam-webster.com/dictionary/resilience. Accessed December 2, 2019.
2. Zurita-Ortega F, Chacón-Cuberos R, Cofre-Bolados C, et al. Relationship of resilience, anxiety and injuries in footballers: Structural equations analysis. PLoS One 2018;13(11):e0207860.
3. Rainey E, Petrey LB, Reynolds M, et al. Psychological factors predicting outcome after traumatic injury: the role of resilience. Am J Surg 2014;208(4):517–23.
4. Harms PD, Brady L, Wood D, et al. Resilience and well-being. In: Diener E, Oishi S, Tay L, editors. Handbook of well-being. Salt Lake City (UT): DEF Publishers; 2018. p. 3–8.
5. Palagini L, Moretto U, Novi M, et al. Lack of resilience is related to stress-related sleep reactivity, hyperarousal, and emotion dysregulation in insomnia disorder. J Clin Sleep Med 2018;14(5):759–66.
6. Whatnall MC, Patterson AJ, Siew YY, et al. Are psychological distress and resilience associated with dietary intake among australian university students? Int J Environ Res Public Health 2019;16(21):4099.
7. Li Y, Bates TC. You can't change your basic ability, but you work at things, and that's how we get hard things done: testing the role of growth mindset on response to setbacks, educational attainment, and cognitive ability. J Exp Psychol 2019;148(9):1640–55.

8. Shanaleft T, Hasn O, Dyrbye L, et al. Changes in burnout and satisfaction with work-life balance in physicians and the general US working population between 2011 and 2014. Mayo Clin Proc 2015;90(12):1600–13.
9. Shanafelt T, Hasan O, Dyrbye LN, et al. Changes in burnout and satisfaction with work-life balance in physicians and the general US working population between 2011 and 2014. Mayo Clin Proc 2015;90(12):1600–13.
10. Aujla I, Farrer R. The role of psychological factors in the career of the independent dancer. Front Psychol 2015;6:1688–2015.
11. Smith B, Dalen J, Wiggins K, et al. The brief resilience scale: assessing the ability to bounce back. Int J Behav Med 2008;15(3):194–200.
12. Sinclair V, Wallston K. The development and psychometric evaluation of the Brief Resilient Scale. Assessment 2004;11(1):94–101.
13. Belo P, Pocinho R, Rodrigues J, et al. Testing the BRCS structure through a multi-group analysis. Res Psychol Behav Sci 2016;4(1):15–8.
14. Lopez-Pina JA, Meseguer-Henarejos AB, Gascón-Cánovas JJ, et al. Measurement properties of the brief resilient coping scale in patients with systemic lupus erythematosus using Rasch analysis. Health Qual Life Outcomes 2016;14:128.
15. Allen N, Nevill A, Brooks J, et al. Ballet injuries: injury incidence and severity over 1 year. J Orthop Sports Phys Ther 2012 Sep;42(9):781–90.
16. Seligman M. Penn Resiliency Program. Available at: https://ppc.sas.upenn.edu/services/penn-resilience-training. Accessed January 12, 2020.
17. Brunwasser S, Gillham JE, Kim ES, et al. A meta-analytic review of the Penn Resiliency Program's effect on depressive symptoms. J Consult Clin Psychol 2009;77(6):1042–54.
18. Spry D. Cognitive behavioural coaching pocketbook. Hants (England): Management Pocketbooks Ltd; 2010.
19. Centre for Clinical Interventions. Module 6: Perfectionism in Perspective. Available at: https://www.cci.health.wa.gov.au/~/media/CCI/Consumer%20Modules/Perfectionism%20in%20Perspective/Perfectionism%20in%20Perspective%20-%2006%20-%20Challenging%20my%20perfectionistic%20thinking.pdf. Accessed January 12, 2020.
20. Strecher VJ. On purpose: lessons in life and health from the Frog, Dung Beetle, and Julia. Ann Arbor (MI): Dung Beetle Press; 2013.
21. Williams G, Deci E. Internalization of biopsychosocial values by medical students. J Pers Soc Psychol 1996;70:767–79.
22. Niemiec C, Ryan R, Deci E. Self-determination therapy and the facilitation of intrinsic motivation, social development, and well-being. Am Psychol 2000;55(1):68–78.
23. Shan G. Comparison of repetitive movements between ballet dancers and martial artists: risk assessment of muscle overuse injuries and prevention strategies. Res Sports Med 2005;13(1):63–76.
24. Weiss DS, Shah S, Burchette RJ. A profile of the demographics and training characteristics of professional modern dancers. J Dance Med Sci 2008;12(2):41–6.
25. Fietze I, Strauch J, Holzhausen M, et al. Sleep quality in professional ballet dancers. Chronobiol Int 2009;26(6):1249–62.

Nutritional Concerns for the Artistic Athlete

Dan Benardot, PhD, DHC, RD, LD[a,b]

KEYWORDS

- Artistic athlete nutrition • Aesthetic body composition • Dancer nutrition
- Within-day energy balance • RED-S

KEY POINTS

- Sustaining within-day energy balance is key to optimizing body composition.
- Low-calorie diets are associated with proportionately higher fat mass and lower lean mass.
- Vitamin and mineral supplementation should be undertaken only under the supervision of a medical professional.
- Injury risks are higher in artistic athletes who experience relative energy deficiency.
- A supportive training environment is necessary to enable the desired food-first approach for satisfying nutritional needs.

INTRODUCTION

Artistic athletes practice and/or perform nearly every day, face extreme competition, and are at risk for experiencing an injury that potentially is career ending.[1] Performing artists typically live hectic lifestyles that make satisfying nutritional needs difficult. The resultant infrequent eating patterns can lead to severe fluctuations in energy balance and blood sugar that result in excess body fat and weight gain, leading to an even greater restrictive eating pattern. Artistic athletes often have energy intakes that are 70% to 80% of the recommended intake because of the belief that this strategy will succeed in helping to achieve body weight and aesthetic appearance goals.[2] This nonscience belief occurs often with quick-fix solutions to help resolve nutrient inadequacy through the intake of high-dose supplements or achieving weight goals through severely energy-deficient diets.[3] These behaviors often are due to poor knowledge of nutrition and modeling of poor nutritional habits of admired performers. It also may result from traditional nutritional behaviors in the arts that are perpetuated over many generations as the student becomes the coach. These practices have undesirable outcomes, with a significant proportion lost weight from muscle, bone, and organ

[a] Center for the Study of Human Health, Candler Library, Emory University, Suite 107, Atlanta, GA 30323, USA; [b] Emeritus, Georgia State University, Atlanta, GA, USA
E-mail address: dan.benardot@emory.edu

Phys Med Rehabil Clin N Am 32 (2021) 51–64
https://doi.org/10.1016/j.pmr.2020.09.008
1047-9651/21/© 2020 Elsevier Inc. All rights reserved.

mass as the body makes a perfectly logical survival adaptation in trying to lower the need for energy when insufficient energy is provided.[4] The inevitable weight cycling that occurs induces multiple nutritionally related complications that have a negative impact on both performance and health. It is common for inadequate energy intake and poorly distributed energy substrates to lower power and endurance from the loss of muscle or from poorly stored fuel. In addition, because food is the carrier of vitamins and minerals in addition to energy, inadequate food consumption has a negative impact on the immune system and increases disease risk, increases skeletal injury risk from a loss of bone mineral density, and over time can increase risk of cardiovascular and renal disease.[5] The use of dietary supplements is widespread in the artistic athlete community, with the belief that this strategy enhances nutritional status and lowers nutritional risks.[6] There is increasingly strong evidence, however, that providing high doses of nutrients does not optimally satisfy nutritional needs, because cells prefer smaller regularly delivered doses associated with frequently consumed meals.[7] This article reviews nutritional concerns of artistic athletes, with an emphasis on nutritional strategies that emphasize established scientific nutritional guidelines.

- Consumption of a wide variety of foods is critical for assuring exposure to all necessary vitamins, minerals, phytonutrients, and energy substrates. Monotonous intakes induce malnutrition, because limiting food variety limits nutrient exposure. As an added benefit, consuming a wide variety of foods also helps limit a potentially toxic substance associated with any individual food from causing cellular damage.
- The goal is to provide tissues with just the right amount of energy and nutrients. This is contradictory to the common belief that if a little bit of a nutrient is good for you, more must be better. More than enough is not better than enough.
- The body works in real time, so nutrient and energy intake must dynamically satisfy tissue needs in real time. An automobile gas tank never would be overfilled, even if the distance to be traveled requires 3 tanks of gas. Also, the tank would not be allowed to go to empty. Similarly, the cell should never be overfilled and should never be allowed to get to empty. This requires an eating pattern for an active person to be more frequent with meals that are smaller and dynamically match energy and nutrient utilization.

ENERGY INTAKE AND ENERGY BALANCE
Energy Intake

Energy intake is a function of the amounts of carbohydrate, protein, and fat consumed. Artistic athletes may fail in consuming sufficient energy from foods and poorly distribute the energy substrates, with excessive focus on protein and a diminished focus on carbohydrate.[8] It was found that dancers have an energy consumption that is less than half their predicted requirements.[9,10] For artistic athletes to lead healthy lives and successful careers, it is important to consume an appropriate amount and distribution of the 3 macronutrients.

Carbohydrate foods provide a flexible fuel for both the central nervous system and lean tissues that can be metabolized both aerobically and anaerobically and are associated with a wide variety of vitamins and minerals. Assuring adequate carbohydrate consumption to sustain normal blood sugar also is an important factor in sleep, which influences the immune system and promotes exercise recovery and performance.[11] A failure to supply an adequate level of carbohydrate to sustain glycogen stores and blood sugar results in poor mental function and early fatigue. This failure initiates a higher cortisol production that catabolizes muscle to convert muscle-based glucogenic amino acids to glucose so as to assure normal central nervous system function.[12]

Although protein can be metabolized as a source of fuel, this is not its primary function. Ideally, protein should provide sufficient levels of essential amino acids for tissue development and maintenance, including the production of hormones and enzymes, critical for body function. Using protein for fuel, however, elevates the excretion of nitrogenous waste, resulting in greater risk of dehydration and lower bone mineral density.[13] The common overemphasis for protein consumption makes it inevitable that a proportion of the protein consumed will be used to supply energy, a common problem with ketogenic diets.[14]

Fats are a concentrated source of energy that can be metabolized oxidatively and deliver fat-soluble vitamins and essential fatty acids. Different fat sources provide different fatty acids, some of which, like omega-3 fatty acids, are associated with reduced inflammation.[15] Fat is the most concentrated source of energy and, despite its poor reputation, is necessary for health.[16] Excess carbohydrate and/or protein are converted to fat that subsequently can be accessed as a fuel. The storage of carbohydrate and protein to fat, however, is a 1-way metabolic pathway, and once converted cannot be reverse engineered to their original forms. Therefore, the goal for food consumption always should be to satisfy tissue requirements with appropriate distribution and volume of each of the energy substrates without providing too much or too little.

The generally recommended intake range for physically active individuals is 1.2 g/kg/d to 2.0 g/kg/d for protein; 5g/kg/d to 12 g/kg/d for carbohydrate; and sufficient energy from fat to satisfy total energy needs, with the goal of not exceeding 35% of total calories.[17] These daily goals must be delivered in a way that satisfies tissue requirements before, during, and after physical activity. Muscle building and maintenance are complex, involving an appropriate intake of micronutrients, energy balance, and protein. Protein should be consumed in relatively small amounts throughout the day with 20 g to 30 g (80–120 kcal) per meal.[18] The increased protein and meal frequency are associated with significant decreases in total body and abdominal fat.[19] The ingestion of more than 30 g of protein in a single meal does not further enhance muscle protein synthesis.[20,21] One simple strategy to determine how to best protein consumption is as follows.

Example for a 125-lb (57-kg) artistic athlete who wishes to increase muscle mass:

1. Determine daily requirement: 2 g × 57 kg/d = 114 g of protein/d
2. Determine optimal protein distribution: 114 g/20 g per meal = approximately 6 meals/d with 20 g of protein at each meal (example: 1, breakfast; 2, midmorning snack; 3, lunch; 4, midafternoon snack; 5, dinner; and 6, evening snack).

The additional benefits of this eating pattern include maintained normal blood sugar, reduction in fat storage, and maintenance of energy balance throughout the day. Specific planning and cooperation with rehearsal and performance sites to enable multiple opportunities for food storage and provision likely are necessary. The alternative, however, which may result in poor energy balance and consumption of fast foods, can increase tissue inflammation and induce a feeling of sluggishness.[22]

Energy Balance

Energy balance represents the ratio between energy consumed and energy expended and is an essential consideration for achieving the desired aesthetic appearance and the demands of training, performance, and recovery. A severe negative energy balance (ie, greater expenditure than consumption) is a concern, particularly during training periods, because this can have a negative impact on sleep, hormonal balance, and performance and increase injury and obesity risk.[11,23] This failure to adequately consume sufficient energy to sustain a good state of energy balance is referred to as relative energy deficiency in sport (RED-S).[24]

Energy balance traditionally is assessed in 24-hour periods, but assessing within-day energy balance is important. Cheerleaders spending more hours in a negative energy balance had significantly higher body fat percentage than those with less time spent in a negative energy balance.[25] A study assessing energy balance and injuries in ballet dancers found a significant association between injury frequency and energy balance deficits exceeding −400 kcal. It also was found that it was common for ballet dancers to experience this level of energy balance deficits during normal training days.[26] Several studies of male and female athletes have found that sustaining an negative energy balance exceeding −300 calories, even if 24-hour energy balance is satisfied, creates multiple problems that include lower resting metabolic rate (RMR), higher body fat percent, lower estrogen-to-cortisol ratio in female athletes, and lower testosterone-to-cortisol ratio in male athletes.[27–29] The low RMR makes it difficult to accurately predict energy balance, requiring that other indicators of energy balance risk, including serum cortisol, and testosterone or estrogen be measured in at risk artistic athletes.[30]

Female artistic athletes with menstrual disorders often have RED-S with associated lower musculature, higher risk of anemia, lower bone mineral density, and a high eating disorder risk.[31] Although eating disorders are more prevalent in female ballet dancers, anorexia nervosa in male ballet dancers also is of concern.[32] The lower RMR associated with the lower estrogen in female athletes and lower testosterone in male athletes makes it more difficult for the artistic athlete to burn consumed calories, increasing obesity risk. The higher weight results in a continual lowering of food consumption that causes energy metabolism to become increasingly down-regulated.[33]

Ballet dancers with menstrual disorders, compared with other female athletes, have high testosterone and high luteinizing hormone–to–follicle-stimulating hormone ratios.[34] These differences likely are due to inhibited conversion of testosterone to estradiol, which is associated with inadequate energy intake of below 30 kcal/kg fat-free mass/d.[35] Amenorrhoeic ballet dancers were found to be interested in learning about personal calories expended and body composition but were poorly compliant in providing information on foods consumed and body image, a behavior suggestive of an eating disorder.[36] Female ballet dancers who had energy metabolism assessed before and after ballet performance had significantly increased appetite stimulating hormone ghrelin postperformance, but energy intake remained below the estimated requirement because of caloric restriction.[37] These problems, however, are not inevitable, because a 9-month nutritional intervention successfully changed energy and nutrient intakes, restoring normal menses.[38]

Because of the high energy/nutrient requirements associated with growth and physical activity, it is important for young dancers to avoid RED-S during this important developmental window.[39] Adolescent ballet dancers have multiple nutritionally related issues associated with inadequate energy consumption that include delayed menarche, which is associated with low bone mineral density; high risk for eating disorder; and low bone mineral density of trabecular bone, including the lumbar spine and femoral neck.[40] In addition, sustaining an energy deficit state during a performance can result in breakdown of lean mass and increased fat mass.[41] These findings suggest that early identification and intervention of artistic athletes who are at risk for RED-S will result in significant health and performance benefits.

HYDRATION

The goal of good hydration, which is critical for health and performance, is to sustain an optimal hydration state rather than to recover from underhydration. A failure to sustain euhydration results in lower blood volume, which lowers the sweat rate and cardiac stroke volume; elevated body temperature from inability to dissipate exercise-associated heat through sweat; greater rate of blood sugar and glycogen use, which is associated with early fatigue; and poor central nervous system function that has a negative impact on coordination and function.[17,42] Fluid loss exceeding 2% of body weight has a negative impact on both mental acuity and exercise performance.[43] Dehydration risk can be diminished as follows[44]: assessing the sense of thirst first thing in the morning and observing urine color (greater thirst and darker urine both suggest underhydration); drinking ample quantities of water when consuming foods; determining weight loss from before and after training and increasing fluid consumption during training to limit loss to less than 2% body weight (1 lb of weight loss = 16 oz of fluid); and developing a strategy that enables frequent beverage sipping during both training and performance.

Because blood sugar and blood volume both are reduced during physical activity when sweat rates increase, the goal of a sports beverage is to replace what is lost to sustain normalcy by providing water, salt, and sugar. Sustaining blood sugar during training inhibits the breakdown of muscle and enables better central nervous system and muscle function.[17] Learning how to drink the sports beverage through frequent sipping is better than waiting for thirst and drinking a large volume for recovery.[45]

During the period prior to training or performance, artistic athletes can consume approximately 8.8 mL fluid/kg (approximately 12 oz for a 100-lb person) or more, with the goal of creating relatively clear urine and providing enough time for excess fluid to be excreted via urine.[46] Consumption of adequate fluid prior to training or performance is better enabled if artistic athletes always have fluid with them.[46] Because the thirst sensation does not occur until approximately 1.5 L of body water already has been lost, thirst should not be relied on as an indicator of when to drink. Occasionally sipping on a sports beverage during this period helps assure that the artistic athlete will begin training with normal blood sugar and normal blood volume, both of which contribute to an enhanced training benefit.[17] It also is important that no alcoholic beverage be consumed during the pretraining period, because alcohol creates diuresis, with greater fluid volume lost than consumed.[47]

Artistic athletes who consume fluids during training can experience reduced fatigue and lower risk of muscular injury. Conversely, underhydration results in early onset fatigue.[17,48] Ideally, time is spent to find an appropriately constituted and well-tolerated sports beverage. Well-tolerated sports beverages typically have sodium concentrations in the range of 100 mg/cup to 200 mg/cup and multiple carbohydrate sources that create a 6% to 7% carbohydrate solution. Beverages containing both sucrose and glucose rather than glucose only are both performance enhancing and well tolerated.[49]

The volume of carbohydrate provided during exercise is an important consideration, because providing too much too fast may induce gastrointestinal distress. The stop-and-start nature of artistic athlete training suggests that an intake of approximately 30-g carbohydrate/h is desirable. To put this into perspective, 8 oz (1 cup) of a typical sports beverage provides 14 g of carbohydrate (56 calories), suggesting that sipping on a 16-oz bottle of sports beverage over the course of a 2.5-hour training session should satisfy carbohydrate needs adequately and normalize blood volume.[17]

Recovery after training is an important consideration, because physical activity likely results in more fluid lost via sweat than is replaced, even when well-designed hydration practices are followed.[50] As fluids continue to be lost postexercise, more fluid should be consumed during the postexercise period than the fluid volume that was lost during exercise.[51] Performing artists should have ready fluids and carbohydrate snacks to consume immediately postexercise to quickly normalize the hydration state and also recover glycogen stores. A small amount of good-quality protein (approximately 10 g) also should be consumed immediately postexercise as part of the recovery strategy to enhance muscle recovery and reduce muscle soreness.[52]

VITAMINS AND MINERALS

Vitamins and minerals are essential micronutrients that aid in maintaining cells, tissues, organs, and other processes essential to life. Individuals consuming a balanced and varied diet that satisfies energy needs are likely also to satisfy vitamin and mineral needs. Because many artistic athletes are on restrictive intakes, however, vitamin and mineral intakes may be at risk. Young female ballet dancers had consumption levels that were greater than 60% below the recommended intake level for calcium, folate, magnesium, and selenium, and approximately 30% had below-normal serum iron values for hemoglobin and ferritin.[53] Young female ballet dancers, compared with same-age female non–ballet dancers, consumed less energy, had lower lean mass, and had insufficient intakes multiple minerals/vitamins.[54] Vegetarians also are at greater risk of inadequate vitamin B_{12}, vitamin D, omega-3 fatty acids, calcium, and zinc. Although it certainly is possible, with diligence and knowledge, to be a vegan or vegetarian and receive all of the needed energy and nutrients from consumed foods, it is easier to obtain these nutrients from a more varied diet.[55] Seasonal variation in vitamin consumption also is an important consideration. Elite ballet dancers who supplemented with vitamin D during the reduced sunlight exposure of winter had better muscular performance and reduced injury occurrence.[56]

An assessment of aesthetic athletes has found that food-derived vitamin and mineral deficiencies were common, with the greatest risk for inadequacy for phosphorus, vitamin A, niacin, and zinc.[57] A survey of dancers (9% aged 35–44 y; 31% aged 24–34 y; and 60% aged 16–24 y) found that 69% were consuming nutritional supplements, and the majority had suffered muscular injuries, with most in the lower back, lower legs, and feet.[9] A recent survey found that most dancers, regardless of gender or dance discipline, consumed nutritional supplements without guidance.[6] The International Olympic Committee consensus statement on dietary supplements makes it clear that professional guidance is strongly advised before taking dietary supplements and that a food-first approach to satisfying nutritional needs is recommended.[7] Arbitrary intake of vitamin and mineral supplements, taken without guidance and without a clear biological need to help reverse a specific nutrient deficiency, may create more problems than are resolved and may provide a false sense of security that nutrient needs are satisfied.

The primary vitamin and mineral concerns include vitamin D, calcium, and iron.[17] Iron deficiency, with and without anemia, is the most common nutrient deficiency in athletes and in normally menstruating women, resulting in fatigue, lower infection resistance, poor muscle function, poor ability to concentrate, and low-energy metabolism.[58] Regular and intense training has been shown to increase blood loss and hemolysis of red blood cells, and it has been estimated that this may raise the minimum iron requirement for activities of higher intensity by 30%.[59] Maintaining good iron status is a significant health and performance concern for artistic athletes. A study assessing the association between muscular strength and iron status (serum hemoglobin, hematocrit, and ferritin) found a significantly positive association in normal iron status compared with female dancers with iron deficiency.[60] Ideally, artistic athletes should have regular annual blood test to determine iron status before considering taking iron supplements, because taking supplemental iron in the wrong amounts and the wrong times may have a negative impact on the absorption of other divalent minerals (calcium, zinc, and magnesium) and may cause intestinal damage.[61]

Vitamin D has multiple functions, including absorption of calcium, improved immune function, and enhanced muscle recovery. A deficiency of vitamin D has clear performance implications, with increased risk of stress fracture, bone/joint injury, overtraining injury, and elevated muscle pain with associated muscular weakness.[62] Food sources of vitamin D include eggs, fatty fish and fish liver oil, sun-exposed mushrooms, and fortified dairy products. Achieving satisfactory vitamin D status is difficult because artistic athletes spend most training and performing time indoors, inhibiting adequate ultraviolet light exposure. A study of basketball players found a strong association between the lower sunlight exposure associated with indoor practice and lower bone mineral density.[63] Because vitamin D levels of commonly consumed foods may not satisfactorily provide sufficient vitamin D and artistic athletes have limited sun exposure as a result of the many hours of indoor training, this vitamin presents a clear case where supervised vitamin D supplementation may be warranted following an examination of serum vitamin D.[64]

Calcium is essential for bone and tooth structure, blood clotting, nerve transmission, and pH control. The buffering action of excess supplemental calcium may interfere with protein digestion, which requires an acidic gastric pH.[65] Excess calcium intake also may interfere with the absorption of other divalent minerals (zinc, iron, and magnesium) if consumed at the same time.[66] To avoid this competitive absorption possibility, calcium supplements should not be taken at the same time as an iron-containing meal or supplement. Good food sources of calcium include dairy products, dark green vegetables, bean, and peas. The high oxalic acid presence in dark green vegetables limits the absorption of both iron and calcium from these foods.[67] Briefly dipping vegetables into boiling water (ie, blanching), however, diminishes the oxalic acid content and enhances absorption. It should be considered that nutrients work together, so even an adequate calcium intake that is associated with a vitamin D deficiency results in calcium deficiency.

WEIGHT AND BODY COMPOSITION

Weight is a measure of total mass whereas body composition measures major body tissues that differentiate between fat mass and fat-free mass. Fat mass refers to the total weight of fat, whereas fat-free mass refers to any body tissue that is not fat, including lean mass, skeletal mass, and body water.[27] Maintaining a healthy weight and body composition largely results from sustaining real-time energy balance, appropriate nutrient intake, proper hydration, and adequate rest.[17] Artistic athletes must fulfill 2 important goals, including sustaining a body composition that can contribute to performance and achieving a specific aesthetic appearance. Assessment of body composition is important for artistic athletes because they have high rates of eating disorders, energy restriction, and inadequate nutrient intake, and they are known to participate in harmful eating behaviors, like binge-eating and purging behaviors.[68,69]

Feedback provided to the artistic athlete should be provided in terms that promote positive action. For instance, telling an artistic athlete that his/her body fat percent is high may result is restrictive eating, regardless of other communicated strategies.

Using the inverse of this value, however, lean mass percent, and informing artistic athletes that they need to increase musculature may well increase the success of the intervention. Trend data on any individual are needed to better understand if an intervention is necessary. An artistic athlete with low percent lean mass may have had an even lower value 1 month earlier, suggesting that an effective strategy already has been implemented. Proposing an intervention to this artistic athlete may interfere with a strategy that already is working, emphasizing the critical importance of trend monitoring in this population.

AGE AND GENDER

Child performers are going through a growth period that requires more energy and nutrients to sustain normal growth and development. This, coupled with the demands of physical activity, mandates a high level of planning to assure adequate eating opportunities of nutritious foods and beverages. The American Academy of Pediatrics has clear guidance on promoting healthy weight-control practices in young athletes, including avoidance of rapid weight change, assuring that weight gain is primarily lean mass, that weight loss is primarily fat mass, and that the focus should be the appropriate intakes of foods and beverages rather than supplements.[70]

Compared with younger athletes, older artistic athletes are more likely to take longer to recover from a training session, typically have lower bone mineral density, and may have gastrointestinal tract functional changes, decreasing absorption for certain nutrients. Although younger and older athletes can increase lean mass at the same rate, older athletes can lose lean mass significantly faster if muscles are not used.[71] This makes avoidance of RED-S especially important in this population, because a well-distributed eating pattern is more likely to avoid malabsorption and muscle loss issues.

Female performers are at particularly high risk of altering reproductive hormones and stress hormones with RED-S, which has multiple negative impacts on bone and muscle health and central nervous system function.[17,24,71] Because of menstrual losses, female athletes are more likely than male athletes to develop iron deficiency and iron deficiency anemia, placing an elevated importance on consuming foods that are good iron sources.[72] Female artistic athletes also are at risk of menstrual dysfunction. Appropriately consumed energy/nutrient intake, however, typically is sufficient to reverse menstrual dysfunction and stop the associated reduction in bone mass.[31]

SUMMARY

It has been observed that the energy deficits and RED-S often seen in artistic athletes are attributable mainly to inadequate dietary planning, and there is evidence that increased planning and nutrition education have a positive impact on food intake.[73] Importantly, those at greatest risk for adopting abnormal eating behaviors appear to benefit the most from nutrition intervention.[74,75] Optimizing nutritional status requires planning equal to the attention that goes into training and rehearsals. Achieving a good nutritional status is more likely if the rehearsal studio enables the provision and/or storage of healthy meals, snacks, and beverages that can be made available to performers before, during, and after training/rehearsals. Each period of training has different nutritional demands, with the pretraining food consisting of a high level of low-fiber carbohydrate, moderate protein, low-fat foods, and hydration beverages, and the post-training period consisting of recovery fluids, replacement carbohydrates, and high-quality proteins.[17]

Overtraining syndrome often can be attributed to insufficient carbohydrate intake or poor hydration and is likely to result in poor performance and increased injury risk.[76] It is important that artistic athletes recognize the early signs of overtraining syndrome, which includes muscle soreness, decreased vigor, loss of appetite, and inability to perform at the previous training load.[74] Overuse injuries are most likely to occur if the training causes repetitive stress to bone and muscles at a rate greater than the tissues can be repaired.[77] Consumption of good-quality protein, carbohydrate, and fluids soon after training ends will enable improved recovery from tissue stress that occurs during training.[17]

When not physically active, it is recommended to maintain energy intake every 3 hours to avoid blood sugar dropping and losing lean mass. Low blood sugar also is likely to result in an elevated insulin response, regardless of what eventually is consumed, encouraging fat gain and overeating.[78,79] When physically active, the reduction in blood sugar to below the normal range can occur much more quickly, which can be mitigated by sipping on a sports beverage during training. This sipping strategy has the combined benefit of maintaining both blood sugar and blood volume. Premature fatigue commonly occurs when athletes experience dehydration and/or depletion of carbohydrate stores.[80]

For the first 4 hours after training, the consumption of 1.0 g/kg/h to 1.2 g/kg/h of carbohydrates and 10 g of protein/h should be consumed to aid recovery.[17] It is not uncommon for artistic athletes to engage in large meal consumption after training and/or performance. This postloading strategy typically is followed because an insufficient level of energy was consumed prior to the training/performance but is not the optimal strategy for sustaining musculature and minimizing fat gain.[81]

CONCLUSION

Nutrition and physical activity are integrated factors that should be well planned to obtain the desired health, performance, and appearance benefits. Restricted energy intakes are associated with multiple problems, including loss of lean mass, hormonal alterations, loss of bone mineral density, longer exercise recovery, and increased injury risk. Using body weight as a criterion for determining nutritional adequacy is suboptimal, because it fails to differentiate between the relative loss or gain of different body tissues, including lean mass, fat mass, and bone mass. Although carbohydrate often is viewed as an inferior energy substrate for active individuals, it almost always is the limiting substrate in performance. In many cases, the excess focus on protein naturally diminishes the intake of carbohydrates below optimal levels. Although all nutrients are important, artistic athletes often fail to consume them in a way that will achieve the desired appearance and performance outcomes. Protein, for instance, is best consumed in relatively small amounts that are well distributed throughout the day and while in a good state of energy balance. Sustaining a good state of hydration throughout the day is critical for both health and performance. Ideally, appropriate planning will enable artistic athletes to pursue a nutritional strategy that encourages consumption of whole foods and discourages the arbitrary use of dietary supplements. There is no substitute for consuming the right foods and beverages of the right kinds, in the right amounts, and at the right times.

CLINICS CARE POINTS

- 'Weight' and 'BMI' may be misleading metrics as they fail to differentiate between the constituents of weight. Assessing change in lean, bone, and fat mass provides more clinically useful information.

- The traditional 24-hour "Calories In and Calories Out" assessment of energy balance adequacy fails to assess risk of significant real-time energy balance deficiency.
- The distribution of protein consumption throughout the day is an important factor in satisfying protein needs.
- The limiting substrate in performance is more likely to be carbohydrate than protein, yet the focus is commonly protein.
- Artistic athletes experience a fast lowering of blood sugar, and lose water and electrolytes (primarily sodium chloride) in sweat during rehearsal and performance. Drinking water alone during these times does not satisfy hydration needs.
- A 'food-first' approach is a better strategy for satisfying nutritional needs than an overreliance of nutrient supplements. This requires meal and snack planning, and a supportive rehearsal/performance environment.

ACKNOWLEDGEMENT

To the students in 'Nutrition for the Performing Arts' class at Emory University, whose creativity contributed to the writing of this paper.

DISCLOSURE

The author has nothing to disclose.

REFERENCES

1. Dick RW, Berning JR, Dawson W, et al. Athletes and the arts-The role of sports medicine in the performing arts. Curr Sports Med Rep 2013;12(6):397–403.
2. Koutedakis Y, Jamurtas A. The dancer as a performing athlete. Sports Med 2004; 34(10):651–61.
3. Thompson C. Get fit quick? The pitfalls of the latest health trends. Dance Magazine 2014;31–3.
4. Duloo AG, Montani JP. Dieting and cardiometabolic risks. Obes Rev 2015; 16(suppl 1):1–6.
5. Montani JP, Schutz Y, Duloo AG. Dieting and weight cycling as risk factors for Cardiometabolic diseases: who is really at risk? Obes Rev 2015;16(Suppl 1):7–18.
6. Zaletel P. Knowledge and use of nutritional supplements in different dance disciplines. Phys Educ Sport 2019;17(3):619–32.
7. Maughan RJ, Burke LM, Dvorak J, et al. IOC consensus statement: dietary supplements and the high-performance athlete. Br J Sports Med 2018;52: 439–55.
8. Manore MM, Patton-Lopez MM, Wong SS. Sports nutrition knowledge, behaviors and beliefs of high school soccer players. Nutrients 2017;9:350.
9. Pacy P, Khalouha M, Koutedakis Y. Body composition, weight control and nutrition in dancers. Dance Res 1996;14(2):93–105.
10. Kazarez M, Cristóbal RV, Ros FE. Perception and distortion of body image in Spanish women dancers based on academic year and age. Nutr Hosp 2018; 35:661–8.
11. Doherty R, Madigan S, Warrington G, et al. Sleep and nutrition interactions: Implications for athletes. Nutrients 2019;11:822.

12. Mor A, Kayacan Y, Ipekoglu G, et al. Effect of carbohydrate-electrolyte consumption on insulin, cortisol hormones and blood glucose after high-intensity exercise. Arch Physiol Biochem 2019;125(4):344–50.

13. Ozkan I, Ibrahim CH. Dehydration, skeletal muscle damage and inflammation before the competitions among the elite wrestlers. J Phys Ther Sci 2016;28:162–8.

14. Cooper R, Naclerio F, Allgrove J, et al. Effects of a carbohydrate and caffeine gel on intermittent sprint performance in recently trained males. Pediatr Exerc Sci 2014;14(4):353–61.

15. Heaton LE, Davis JK, Rawson ES, et al. Selected in-season nutritional strategies to enhance recovery for team sport athletes: A practical overview. Sports Med 2017;47:2201–18.

16. Petrie HJ, Stover EA, Horswill CA. Nutritional concerns for the child and adolescent competitor. Nutrition 2004;20(7–8):620–31.

17. Thomas DT, Erdman KA, Burke LM, et al. American College of Sports Medicine Joint Position Statement. Nutrition and Athletic Performance. Med Sci Sports Exerc 2016;48(3):543–68.

18. Burke LM, Jeukendrup AE, Jones AM, et al. Contemporary Nutrition Strategies to Optimize Performance in Distance Runners and Race Walkers. Int J Sport Nutr Exerc Metab 2019;29(2):117–29.

19. Arciero PJ, Ormsbee MJ, Gentile CL, et al. Increased protein intake and meal frequency reduces abdominal fat during energy balance and energy deficit. Obesity 2013;21(7):1357–66.

20. Symons TB, Sheffield-Moore M, Wolfe RR, et al. A Moderate Serving of High-Quality Protein Maximally Stimulates Skeletal Muscle Protein Synthesis in Young and Elderly Subjects. J Am Diet Assoc 2009;109(9):1582–6.

21. Paddon-Jones D, Campbell WW, Jacques PF, et al. Protein and healthy aging. Am J Clin Nutr 2015;101(6):1339s–45s.

22. Stark JH, Neckerman K, Lovasi GS, et al. Neighbourhood food environments and body mass index among New York City adults. J Epidemiol Community Health 2013;67(9):736–42.

23. Brown MA, Howatson G, Quin E, et al. Energy intake and energy expenditure of pre-professional female contemporary dancers. PLoS One 2017;12(2):e0171998.

24. Mountjoy M, Sundgot-Borgen JK, Burke LM, et al. IOC consensus statement on relative energy deficiency in sport (RED-S): 2018 update. Br J Sports Med 2018;52:687–97.

25. Bellissimo MP, Licata AD, Nucci A, et al. Relationships between estimated hourly energy balance and body composition in professional cheerleaders. J Sci Sport Exer 2019;1:69–77.

26. Harrison EC, McCarroll C, Thompson WR, et al. Within-day energy balance and the relationship to injury rates in pre-professional ballet dancers. Atlanta (GA): Thesis-Georgia State University; 2009. Available at: https://scholarworks.gsu.edu/nutrition_theses/7.

27. Deutz R, Benardot D, Martin D, et al. Relationship between energy deficits and body composition in elite female gymnasts and runners. Med Sci Sports Exerc 2000;32(3):659–68.

28. Fahrenholtz I, Sjödin A, Benardot D, et al. Within-day energy deficiency and reproductive function in female endurance athletes. Scand J Med Sci Sports 2018;1(8). https://doi.org/10.1111/sms.13030.

29. Torstveit MK, Fahrenholtz I, Stenqvist TB, et al. Within-day energy deficiency and metabolic perturbation in male endurance athletes. Int J Sport Nutr Exerc Metab 2018;28(4):419–27.

30. Staal S, Sjödin A, Fahrenholtz I, et al. Low RMR ratio as a surrogate marker for energy deficiency, the choice of predictive equation vital for correctly identifying male and female ballet dancers at risk. Int J Sport Nutr Exerc Metab 2018;28: 412–8.

31. Łagowska K, Jeszka J. The evaluation of eating behavior and nutritional status of ballet dncers with menstrual disorders. Med Sport 2011;15(4):213–8.

32. Marra M, Sammarco R, De Filippo E, et al. Resting energy expenditure, body composition, and phase angle in anorectic, ballet dancers and constitutionally lean males. Nutrients 2019;11:502.

33. Myburgh KH, Berman C, Novick I, et al. Decreased resting metabolic rate in ballet dancers with menstrual irregularity. Int J Sport Nutr 1999;9:285–94.

34. Łagowska K, Kapczuk K. Testosterone concentrations in female athletes and ballet dancers with menstrual disorders. Eur J Sport Sci 2016;16(4):490–7.

35. Davis SR, Wahlin-Jacobsen S. Testosterone in women-the clinical significance. Lancet Diabetes Endocrinol 2015. https://doi.org/10.1016/S2213-8587(15)00284-3.

36. Glace B, Kremenic I, Liederbach M. Energy conservation in amenorrheic ballet dancers. Med Probl Perform Art 2006;21:96–104.

37. Kim SY, Cho JH, Lee JH, et al. Changes in body composition, energy metabolism, and appetite-regulating hormones in Korean professional female ballet dancers before and after ballet performance. J Dance Med Sci 2019;23(4):173–80.

38. Łagowska K, Kapczuk K, Jeszka J. Nine month nutritional intervention improves restoration of menses in young female athletes and ballet dancers. J Int Soc Sports Nutr 2014;11(52). https://doi.org/10.1186/s12970-014-0052-9.

39. Brown DD. Nutrition, bone health, and the young dancer. Prevention of Injuries in the Young Dancer. In: Solomon R, Solomon J, Micheli L, editors. Contemporary pediatric and adolescent sports medicine. Cham (Switzerland): Springer; 2017. p. 187–201.

40. Burckhardt P, Wynn E, Krieg M-A, et al. The effects of nutrition, puberty and dancing on bone density in adolescent ballet dancers. J Dance Med Sci 2011; 15(2):51–60.

41. Di Mascio P, Kaiser S, Sies H. Lycopene as the most efficient biological carotenoid singlet oxygen quencher. Arch Biochem Biophys 1989;274(2):532–8.

42. Clarkson P. Nutrition fact sheet: Fueling the Dancer. Int Assoc Dance Med Sci. Available at: www.DanceMedicine.org. Accessed April 10, 2020.

43. Trangmar SJ, González-Alonso J. Heat, Hydration and the Human Brain, Heart and Skeletal Muscles. Sports Med 2019;49(S1):69–85.

44. Casa DJ, DeMartini JK, Berjeron MF, et al. National Athletic Trainers' Association position statement: exertional heat illnesses. J Athl Train 2015;50(9):986–1000.

45. Koutedakis Y. Nutrition to fuel dance: A brief review. Dance Research: J Soc Dance Res 1996;14(2):76–93.

46. Goulet ED. Dehydration and endurance performance in competitive athletes. Nutr Rev 2012;70(Suppl 2):S132–6.

47. Owens DS. Lifestyle modification: diet, exercise, sports, and other issues. In: Naidu S, editor. Hypertrophic cardiomyopathy. Cham (Switzerland): Springer; 2019. p. 169–82. https://doi.org/10.1007/978-3-319-92423-6_12.

48. Burke LM, Castell LM, Casa DJ, et al. International Association of Athletics Federations Consensus Statement 2019: Nutrition for Athletics. Int J Sport Nutr Exerc Metab 2019a;29:73–84.

49. Triplett D, Doyle JA, Rupp JC, et al. An isocaloric glucose-fructose beverage's effect on simulated 100-km cycling performance compared with a glucose-only beverage. Int J Sport Nutr Exerc Metab 2010;20:122–31.

50. Garth AK, Burke LM. What do athletes drink during competitive sporting activities? Sports Med 2013;43(7):539–64.

51. Kenefick RW, Cheuvront SN. Hydration for recreational sport and physical activity. Nutr Rev 2012;70(s2). https://doi.org/10.1111/j.1753-4887.2012.00523.x.

52. Beelen M, Burke LM, Gibala MJ, et al. Nutritional strategies to promote postexercise recovery. Int J Sport Nutr Exerc Metab 2010;20(6):515–32.

53. Beck KL, Mitchell S, Foskett A, et al. Dietary intake, anthropometric characteristics, and iron and vitamin D status of female adolescent ballet dancers living in New Zealand. Int J Sport Nutr Exerc Metab 2015;25:335–43.

54. Kalnióa L, Selga G, Sauka M, et al. Comparison of body composition and energy intake of young female ballet dancers and ordinary school girls. Proc Latv Acad Sci 2017;6(711):423–7.

55. Brown DD. Nutritional considerations for the vegetarian and vegan dancer. J Dance Med Sci 2018;22(1):44–53.

56. Wyon MA, Koutedakis Y, Woman R, et al. The influence of winter vitamin D supplementation on muscle function and injury occurrence in elite ballet dancers: A controlled study. J Sci Med Sport 2014;17(1):8–12.

57. Soric M, Misigoj-Durakovic M, Pedisic Z. Dietary intake and body composition of prepubescent female aesthetic athletes. Int J Sport Nutr Exerc Metab 2008;18: 343–54.

58. Haymes E. Iron. In: Driskell J, Wolinsky I, editors. Sports nutrition: vitamins and trace elements. New York: ©CRC/Taylor & Francis; 2006. p. 203–16.

59. Institute of Medicine, Food and Nutrition Board. Dietary reference intakes (DRIs): vitamin A, vitamin K, Boron, Chromium, Copper, Iodine, Iron, Manganese, Molybdenum, Nickel, Silicon, Vanadium, and Zinc. Washington (DC): National Academy Press; 2001. p. 290–393.

60. Agopyan A, Tekin D. Isokinetic knee muscular strength is associated with hematologic variables in female modern dancers. J Hum Sport Exerc 2018;13(2): 305–18.

61. Schümann K, Ettle T, Szegner B, et al. On risks and benefits of iron supplementation recommendations for iron intake revisited. J Trace Elem Med Biol 2007; 21(3):147–68.

62. Moran DS, McClung JP, Kohen T, et al. Vitamin D and physical performance. Sports Med 2013;43(7):601–11.

63. Bescós García R, Rodrígues Guisado FA. Low levels of vitamin D in professional basketball players after wintertime: Relationship with dietary intake of vitamin D and calcium. Nutr Hosp 2011;26(5):945–51.

64. Rowan FE, Benjamin-Laing H, Kennedy A, et al. Self-directed oral vitamin D supplementation in professional ballet dancers: A randomized controlled trial pilot study. J Dance Med Sci 2019;23(3):91–6.

65. Lewis JR, Zhu K, Prince RL. Adverse events from calcium supplementation: relationship to errors in myocardial infarction self-reporting in randomized controlled trials of calcium supplementation. J Bone Mineral Res 2012;27(3):719–22.

66. Corte-Real J, Bohn T. Interaction of divalent minerals with lipsoluble nutrients and phytochemicals during digestion and influences on their bioavailability-a review. Food Chem 2018;252(30):285–93.
67. Mihrete Y. Review on mineral malabsorption and reducing technologies. Int J Neurol Phys Ther 2019;5(1):25–30.
68. Ringham R, Klump K, Kaye W, et al. Eating disorder symptomatology among ballet dancers. Int J Eat Disord 2006;39(6). https://doi.org/10.1002/eat.20299.
69. Leal LLA, Barbosa GSL, Ferreira RLU, et al. Cross-validaiton of prediction equations for estimating body composition in ballet dancers. PLoS One 2019;14(7): e0219045.
70. Carl RL, Johnson MD, Martin TJ, et al. Promotion of Healthy Weight-Control Practices in Young Athletes. Pediatrics 2017;140(3):e20171871.
71. Desbrow B, Burd NA, Tarnopolsky M, et al. Nutrition for special populations: Young, female, and masters athletes. Int J Sport Nutr Exerc Metab 2019;29: 220–7.
72. Pedlar CR, Brugnara C, Bruinvels G, et al. Iron balance and iron supplementation for the female athlete: A practical approach. Eur J Sport Sci 2018;18(2):295–305.
73. Civil R, Lamb A, Loosmore D, et al. Assessment of dietary intake, energy status, and factors associated with RED-S in vocational female ballet students. Front Nutr 2019;5. https://doi.org/10.3389/fnut.2018.00136. Article 136.
74. Doyle-Lucas AF, Davy BM. Development and evaluation of an educational intervention program for pre-professional adolescent ballet dancers-Nutrition for optimal performance. J Dance Med Sci 2011;15(2):65–75.
75. Yannakoulia M, Sitara M, Matalas A-L. Reported eating behavior and attitudes improvement after a nutrition intervention program in a group of young female dancers. Int J Sport Nutr Exerc Metab 2002;12:24–32.
76. Meeusen R, Duclos M, Gleeson M, et al. Prevention, Diagnosis, and Treatment of the Overtraining Syndrome. Med Sci Sports Exerc 2013;45(1):186–205.
77. Krivickas LS. Anatomical Factors Associated with Overuse Sports Injuries. Sports Med 1997;24(2):132–46.
78. Areta JL, Burke LM, Ross NL, et al. Timing and distribution of protein ingestion during prolonged recovery from resistance exercise alters microfibrillar protein synthesis. J Physiol 2013;591(9):2319–31.
79. Benardot D. Energy thermodynamics revisited: Energy intake strategies for optimizing athlete body composition and performance. Pensar en Movimiento 2013; 11(2):1–14.
80. Sawka MN, Wenger CB, Pandolf KB. Thermoregulatory Responses to Acute Exercise-Heat Stress and Heat Acclimation. In: Terjung R, editor. Comprehensive Physiology. 2011. p. 157–85.
81. Paddon-Jones D, Rasmussen BB. Dietary protein recommendations and the prevention of sarcopenia. Curr Opin Clin Nutr Metab Care 2009;12(1):86–90.

Nutrition Periodization in Dancers

Jatin P. Ambegaonkar, PhD, ATC, OT, CSCS, FIADMS[a],*, Ann F. Brown, PhD, CISSN[b]

KEYWORDS

- Energy • Performance • Performing artists • Food

KEY POINTS

- Nutrition periodization is the strategic and timed intake of nutrients to successfully meet the varying nutritional demands across the annual dance season.
- During preseason (goals: design, rehearse, and train), dancers should consume 3 to 7 g/kg body mass (BM)/d of carbohydrate, 0.8 to 1.3 g/kg BM/d of fat, and 1.2 to 2.5 g/kg BM/d of protein.
- During in-season (goals: one or more daily performances), dancers should consume 5 to 12 g/kg BM/day of carbohydrate, 1.0 to 1.5 g/kg BM/day of fat, and 1.4 to 2.0 g/kg BM/day of protein.
- During postseason (goals: rest and prepare for the next season), dancers should consume 3 to 4 g/kg BM/day of carbohydrate, 1.0 to 1.2 g/kg BM/day of fat, and 1.5 to 2.3 g/kg BM/day of protein.
- Overall, nutrition periodization can support dancers' training goals (eg, to increase strength) over the season, enhance performance during acute events (eg, performing an hour-long dance), and support optimal recovery (eg, maintenance of lean muscle mass).

INTRODUCTION

Dancing is a unique combination of art and sport movement that involves participants to perform physically demanding, yet aesthetically pleasing movements that require extreme ranges of motion, artistic expression, and musicality.[1–5] To perform successfully, dancers should have enhanced fitness capabilities including flexibility, muscular strength, power, cardiovascular endurance, coordination and balance,[5–8] and appropriate energy intakes.[9,10]

Funding: None.
[a] Sports Medicine Assessment Research and Testing (SMART) Laboratory, George Mason University, 201-F, K Johnson Hall, MSN 4E5, 10890 George Mason Circle, Manassas, VA 20110, USA;
[b] Human Performance Laboratory, Department of Movement Sciences, University of Idaho, College of Education Health & Human Sciences, Physical Education Building 104, 875 Perimeter Drive MS 2401, Moscow, ID 83844, USA
* Corresponding author.
E-mail address: jambegao@gmu.edu

Phys Med Rehabil Clin N Am 32 (2021) 65–73
https://doi.org/10.1016/j.pmr.2020.09.001
1047-9651/21/© 2020 Elsevier Inc. All rights reserved.

pmr.theclinics.com

In athletics, the energy demands of the season fluctuate over the year. To address these fluctuations, practitioners in the sports medicine field have long recommended periodizing training[11–13] and more recently nutritional training.[14–18] Periodization is an organized approach to training that involves progressive cycling of various aspects of a training program during a specific period of time.[16] Periodization involves division of training cycles throughout the course of the year, where volume, frequency, intensity, time, and type of training are manipulated to meet the demands of the sport.[16]

Likewise, in the dance medicine and science field, some investigators have described periodizing training loads[19] and how to integrate fitness training[20] into dancers' overall training regimens. However, to the authors' knowledge, little research exists examining nutrition interventions and the role in enhancing dance performance.[21] Inadequate nutrient intake is linked to a variety of health-related issues such as impaired growth and development, decreased coordination and performance, and increased risk for injury.[22,23] Dance is an activity that often begins at a young age, with most dancers beginning to dance as early as 10 to 11 years old.[24] If dietary needs are not being met during critical growth and development years, dancers can present with health issues earlier than other athletic populations due to the nature of when the activity begins. In addition, dance is an aesthetic sport that places additional pressures on physique and body weight.[3,4,9] These pressures inherently can lead to heightened focus on diet and unhealthy eating behaviors such as restrictive eating.[25,26] Restrictive eating may be the simplest solution for the dancer because relatively little published guidance exists provided on how to adjust the diet throughout the various seasons of dance training, performances, and recovery. Some nutrition recommendations exist for dancers,[9] and the International Association for Dance Medicine & Science has published a practical Nutrition Resource Paper guide for dancers.[27] However, these resources do not specifically detail the intricacies of how dietary recommendations fluctuate with the changes over the day and throughout the dance season. Thus a knowledge gap is present in the recommendations for addressing varying nutritional needs in dancers. This gap exists despite several prior investigators[9,15,17] consistently stating that nutrition can be a limiting factor in athletes when training for strength, power, and endurance gains and is sometimes overlooked, as it pertains to the inclusion to the annual training plan.[18,28]

Overall, dancers' energy demands fluctuate across the season. Accordingly, dancers should adapt their nutrition to match their training or performance schedule. However, information about how to periodize nutrition in dancers is lacking. Thus, the authors aim to (1) introduce nutrition periodization concepts and (2) provide recommendations for nutrition periodization in dancers.

Specifically, the authors discuss nutrition periodization for the dancer as a comprehensive approach toward adequate nutrient intake through the cycles of a dance season. After reviewing this article, readers should be able to, from a nutrition periodization perspective, (1) explain nutrition periodization, (2) recognize basic cycles of a dance season, and (3) describe approaches to help maintain adequate nutrition across the dance season. The current article is not a comprehensive review of the literature regarding nutrition periodization. Rather, in agreement with Mota and colleagues[15] the authors bring attention to dancers' specific nutritional concerns and encourage practitioners to proactively consider nutrition as an integral part of their dancers' training programs.

Nutrition Periodization

Jeukendrup[17] defined periodized nutrition as *"the planned, purposeful, and strategic use of specific nutritional interventions to enhance the adaptations targeted by individual exercise sessions or periodic training plans, or to obtain other effects that will enhance performance longer term."*

The term nutritional training is sometimes used to describe the same methods, and these terms can be used interchangeably.[17] Nutrition periodization encompasses everything including the "when," "why," "how," and "what" of eating and drinking.[14] For dancers, this means eating and drinking optimally to support their training and health.[14]

Nutritional Periodization Demands Across Seasons

Dance is a unique activity in that there are a wide variety of genres that all have differing schedules.[1] However, the overarching similarity is that all genres have a pre-, in-, and postseason.[19] Given that energy demands change across a season,[15–17,19] nutrition periodization can help dancers optimize training-driven alterations in performance while also providing them programmed rest and recovery strategies.[15] The following sections detail how to adapt nutritional intake across the entire dance season (ie, preseason, in-season, and offseason).

Preseason

In the current paper, the authors classify preseason as the period of time where dancers engage in regular classes and dance pieces are designed, choreographed, and rehearsed for the purpose of nutrition periodization. Preseason nutrition variations depend greatly on the individual dancers' goals (eg, increase, decrease, or maintain body mass) and also the dance genre (eg, ballet, modern, hip-hop, etc.). Nevertheless, for all dancers and genres, during preseason, they need to have adequate fitness (eg, power, strength, power, and endurance) to adequately prepare the body for numerous performances that occur in-season. This preparation phase includes proper nutrition both to (1) fuel optimal training and subsequent performances and also to (2) maintain optimal body composition to reduce risk of injury and enhance aesthetics during performance. Nutrition plans for dancers should thus be periodized to match the dancers' training demands, body composition, and performance goals.[15]

Previous researchers have found that dance classes, across genres and levels, are of moderate to high physical activity intensity.[29] Still, similar to sports, this intensity is not consistent throughout the entirety of a class due to the different phases, for example, the warmup/preparatory phase and the center/execution phase. Specifically, the warmup/preparatory phase has more low-intensity physical activity, whereas the center/execution phase has more high physical activity intensity.[30,31] Accordingly, to properly fuel the body for dance classes during preseason, the dancer should consider class intensity to determine macronutrient (ie, carbohydrate, protein, and fat) consumption.

In agreement with prior investigators, the authors recommend that the dancer consume between 3 and 7 g/kg body mass (BM)/day of carbohydrate during preseason to maintain glycogen stores throughout the day.[14,15] Dancers should first evaluate the volume and intensity of their training day to decide how to maintain carbohydrate consumption within this recommended range. For example, on low-intensity and -volume days (ie, <2 hours of class/rehearsal time), carbohydrate should be consumed on the lower end of this range (3–5 g/kg BM/d). As intensity and volume progressively increase, carbohydrate consumption should progressively increase to match the increased demands.[15] If the dancers' goal is to increase body mass during preseason, and training intensity and volume are high, carbohydrate should increase to 6 to 7 g/kg BM/d. However, if the goal is to maintain body mass, the dancer should intake slightly lower carbohydrate (4–7 g/kg BM/d) amounts regardless of training intensity and volume.[15]

Protein consumption will also vary depending on body mass goals specifically if the dancer's goal is to reduce weight.[32] As a general range, the authors recommended that dancers should consume 1.2 to 2.5 g/kg BM/d of protein during preseason. In support, higher protein consumption (2.3 g/kg BM/d) has previously been found to optimize body composition index in collegiate dancers during pre- and in-season.[21] If a dancer is trying to optimize body composition (eg, increase lean soft tissue and decrease fat mass) while training load is high, the dancer needs to consume greater than 2.0 g/kg BM/d protein to both improve satiety and attenuate lean mass loss.[33,34] The authors also emphasize quality weight loss via increased protein intake to prevent performance decrements and possible increased injury in the preseason.

Lastly, dietary fat should be relatively low (0.8 1.3 g/kg BM/d) during preseason. If the intensity and volume of training changes from day to day, the higher end of this range is recommended to maintain energy balance.[15] **Fig. 1** shows macronutrient distribution recommendations during preseason based on intensity, volume, and body mass goals.

In-season

The in-season is the peak performance season. During this time, dancers continue to train and participate in rehearsals/classes and perform regularly throughout the week and often multiple times a day.[19] Dance performances are often a higher intensity activity than dance classes and rehearsals.[30] Therefore, nutrition recommendations should be adapted to match the change in intensity and volume (number of performances per day). It is important to note that different dance genres are across this power-strength-endurance continuum (eg, hip-hop dance-modern-ballet), and performances may last for a few minutes (eg, modern dance) or extend into multiple hours (eg, Indian classical dance). Thus nutrition recommendations will vary across dance genres during in-season.

If dance performances are intense and performed multiple times a day, carbohydrate intake should increase to 5 to 12 g/kg BM/d. Dancers should aim to consume carbohydrate at the higher end of this range on days with multiple performances. The carbohydrates should be consumed throughout the day in multiple smaller meals to maintain glycogen stores.

Protein intake should remain relatively the same or slightly decrease from preseason to 1.4 to 2.0 g/kg BM/d. There are slight differences in recommendations for strength/power athletes (1.7–2.0 g/kg BM/d) and endurance athletes (1.2–1.7 g/kg BM/d) in-season due to the differences in body composition goals.[15] Because dance is an aesthetic sport that requires strength, power, and endurance, dancers' protein intake should remain between 1.4 and 2.0 g/kg BM/d during-season to optimize body composition and performance. To allow the dancer to maintain energy balance on days where intensity and volume are high leading to an increase in aid in energy expenditure, dancers should also slightly increase dietary fat intake slightly to 1.0 to 1.5 g/kg BM/d.

Consistent with the preseason, dancers should also adjust nutrient timing throughout the day during the in-season. Nutrient timing can vary greatly depending

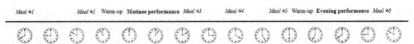

Meal #1   Meal #2 Warm-up Matinee performance Meal #3   Meal #4   Meal #5 Warm-up Evening performance Meal #6

Fig. 1. Macronutrient distribution recommendations during preseason based on intensity, volume, and body mass goals.

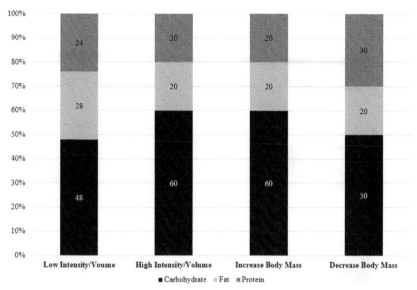

Fig. 2. Example of in-season daily nutrient timing for dancers.

on the dancers' performance schedule. **Fig. 2** depicts an example of a dancer's day and how the dancer may time nutrition intake across the day when multiple performances are scheduled over the day. The intake of nutrition timing is most critical immediately before and after each performance. To provide sufficient energy before a performance, the dancer should consume a meal rich in carbohydrate 10 to 30 minutes (individualized choice) before the performance warm-up.[16] Immediately following a performance, a dancer should consume a meal rich in carbohydrate and protein to replenish glycogen stores and stimulate muscle protein synthesis.[16] Overall, with extreme variations in performance schedules in-season, the dancers are encouraged to consume 4 to 6 smaller meals throughout the day with the emphasis of planning meals around performances.

Postseason
The postseason is often the most challenging time of year for any athlete because of the sudden changes in training schedule. In most cases for the dancer, frequency of dance training decreases substantially and they are typically not taking part in extensive rehearsals or performances. Some dancers may supplement their training regimens with other types of fitness training during this time. However, the postseason recommendations the authors make are based on the assumption that exercise training intensity and volume are significantly reduced in most dancers.

Specifically, carbohydrate intake should be lowered to 3 to 4 g/kg BM/d. This lower range of carbohydrate would suffice for a dancer taking part in supplemental exercise during the postseason. Protein intake should remain high (1.5–2.3 g/kg BM/d) to maintain muscle mass and contribute to satiety during a time of reduced energy expenditure. Dietary fat intake should remain moderate (1.0–1.2 g/kg BM/d) to continue to support proper physiologic function and ensure a healthy entrance into the next preseason.[14] **Fig. 3** describes the overall macronutrient distribution when periodizing nutrition across the seasons for dancers.

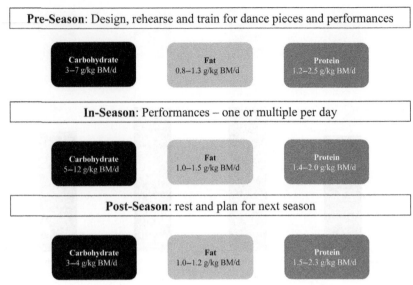

Pre-Season: Design, rehearse and train for dance pieces and performances

Carbohydrate	Fat	Protein
3–7 g/kg BM/d	0.8–1.3 g/kg BM/d	1.2–2.5 g/kg BM/d

In-Season: Performances – one or multiple per day

Carbohydrate	Fat	Protein
5–12 g/kg BM/d	1.0–1.5 g/kg BM/d	1.4–2.0 g/kg BM/d

Post-Season: rest and plan for next season

Carbohydrate	Fat	Protein
3–4 g/kg BM/d	1.0–1.2 g/kg BM/d	1.5–2.3 g/kg BM/d

Fig. 3. Overall macronutrient distribution when periodizing nutrition across the season for dancers.

Special Considerations

Although both sexes participate in dance, nutrition recommendations differ between female and male dancers due to physiologic differences regardless of participation in identical classes, rehearsals, and performances. The menstrual cycle is known to influence performance through changes in metabolism, thermoregulation, and psychological factors.[35] Fluctuations in estrogen and progesterone can lead to increased or decreased performance. Specifically, estrogen is thought to enhance endurance performance through alterations in carbohydrate, fat, and protein metabolism, whereas progesterone may oppose these effects and decrease performance.[36] Of particular concern for the dancer, progesterone peaks in the luteal phase (days 15–28 of a standard 28-day menstrual cycle) and promotes protein breakdown.[36] Therefore, it is suggested to increase protein consumption not only across the dance season but also across menstrual cycle phase, because an irregular or absent menstrual cycle can have negative impacts on the dancers metabolism, performance, and overall health.[37] Thus, female dancers should consider these changes and alter intake appropriately to maintain their energy balance and overall health.

As mentioned earlier, the dance genre will dictate how a dancer trains and performs. However, it is also important to consider the different levels (novice, competition dance, collegiate programs, professional ballet, etc.).[1,19] Collegiate dancers in particular, have a unique challenge in balancing the dance seasons involving dance classes, rehearsals, and performances alongside an academic responsibility and financial strain prevalent in collegiate students.[38] Often at this level (although it is possible at all levels), dancers may find it challenging to follow nutrition recommendations due to the often higher cost of healthy food choices. Consequently, it can be burdensome for them to afford to properly fuel themselves over the dance season. In this case, at the very least, the authors recommend that dancers should consume adequate total calories while attempting to consume macronutrients within the proposed ranges during the different seasons.

SUMMARY

Overall, dancers' energy demands fluctuate over the dance season. Thus they should use nutrition periodization, which is the strategic and timed intake of nutrients to successfully meet these varying nutritional demands across the dance season. Practitioners should use appropriate nutrition periodization over the preseason, in-season, and postseason to support their dancers' training goals over the season. These techniques can help practitioner enhance their dancers' performance during acute events and eventually increase their dancers' career longevity and success.

CONFLICT OF INTEREST

None.

REFERENCES

1. Solomon R, Micheli L. Technique as a consideration in modern dance injuries. Phys Sportsmed 1986;14(8):83–90.
2. Liederbach M. Screening for functional capacity in dancers designing standardized, dance-specific injury prevention screening tools. J Dance Med Sci 1997; 1(3):93–106.
3. Koutedakis Y. Nutrition to Fuel Dance: A Brief Review. Dance Res 1996;14(2): 76–93.
4. Koutedakis Y, Jamurtas T. The Dancer as a Performing Athlete: Physiological Considerations. Sports Med 2004;34:651–61.
5. Angioi M, Metsios G, Koutedakis Y, et al. Physical fitness and severity of injuries in contemporary dance. Med Probl Perform Art 2009;24(1):26–9.
6. Armstrong R, Brogden CM, Milner D, et al. Functional movement screening as a predictor of mechanical loading and performance in dancers. J Dance Med Sci 2018;22(4):203–8.
7. Hincapié CA, Morton EJ, Cassidy JD. Musculoskeletal injuries and pain in dancers: a systematic review. Arch Phys Med Rehabil 2008;89(9):1819–29.
8. Fauntroy V, Nolton E, Ambegaonkar JP. Health-Related Quality of Life (HRQoL) Measures Used in Dance: A Systematic Review. Int J Sports Phys Ther 2020; 15(3):1–10.
9. Sousa M, Carvalho P, Moreira P, et al. Nutrition and nutritional issues for dancers. Med Probl Perform Art 2013;28(3):119–23.
10. Rossiou D, Papadopoulou S, Pagkalos I, et al. Energy expenditure and nutrition status of ballet, jazz and contemporary dance students. Prog Health Sci 2017; 7:31–8.
11. Selye H. Stress and the general adaptation syndrome. Br Med J 1950;1(4667): 1383–92.
12. Rowbottom D. Periodization of training. In: Garrett WE, Kirkendall DR, editors. Exercise and sport science. 1st edition. Philadelphia: Lippincott Williams & Wilkins; 2000. p. 499–511.
13. Frankel CC, Kravitz L. Periodization: latest studies and practical applications. IDEA Pers Train 2000;11(1):15–6.
14. Seebohar B. Nutrition Periodization for Athletes: NSCA Hot Topics. 2018. Available at: http:nsca-lift.org; http://drjj5hc4fteph.cloudfront.net/Articles/Nutrition%20Periodization.pdf. Accessed June 1, 2020.
15. Mota J, Nucklos G, Smith-Ryan A. Nutritional periodization: Applications for the Strength athlete. Strength Cond J 2019;41(5):69–78.

16. Muntaenu AM, Manuc D, Caramoci A, et al. Nutrition timing in top athletes. Med Sport 2014;10(3):2357–63.
17. Jeukendrup AE. Periodized Nutrition for Athletes. Sports Med 2017;47(Suppl 1): 51–63.
18. Stellingwerff T, Morton JP, Burke LM. A Framework for Periodized Nutrition for Athletics. Int J Sport Nutr Exerc Metab 2019;29(2):141–51.
19. Wyon M. Preparing to perform: periodization and dance. J Dance Med Sci 2010; 14(2):67–72.
20. Rafferty S. Considerations for Integrating Fitness into Dance Training. J Dance Med Sci 2010;14(2):45–9.
21. Brown AF, Welsh T, Panton LB, et al. Higher-protein intake improves body composition index in female collegiate dancers. Appl Physiol Nutr Metab Physiol Appl Nutr Metab 2020;45(5):547–54.
22. Loucks AB, Kiens B, Wright HH. Energy availability in athletes. J Sports Sci 2011; 29(Suppl 1):S7–15.
23. Sundgot-Borgen J, Meyer NL, Lohman TG, et al. How to minimise the health risks to athletes who compete in weight-sensitive sports review and position statement on behalf of the Ad Hoc Research Working Group on Body Composition, Health and Performance, under the auspices of the IOC Medical Commission. Br J Sports Med 2013;47(16):1012–22.
24. Storm JM, Wolman R, Bakker EWP, et al. The Relationship Between Range of Motion and Injuries in Adolescent Dancers and Sportspersons: A Systematic Review. Front Psychol 2018;9:287.
25. Robbeson JG, Kruger HS, Wright HH. Disordered Eating Behavior, Body Image, and Energy Status of Female Student Dancers. Int J Sport Nutr Exerc Metab 2015;25(4):344–52.
26. Dwyer J, Eisenberg A, Prelack K, et al. Eating attitudes and food intakes of elite adolescent female figure skaters: a cross sectional study. J Int Soc Sports Nutr 2012;9(1):53.
27. Challis J, Wilson M. Nutrition Resource Paper. 2016. Available at: https://www.iadms.org/page/RPnutrition. Accessed June 2, 2020.
28. Heikura IA, Stellingwerff T, Burke LM. Self-Reported Periodization of Nutrition in Elite Female and Male Runners and Race Walkers. Front Physiol 2018;9:1732.
29. Beck KL, Mitchell S, Foskett A, et al. Dietary Intake, Anthropometric Characteristics, and Iron and Vitamin D Status of Female Adolescent Ballet Dancers Living in New Zealand. Int J Sport Nutr Exerc Metab 2015;25(4):335–43.
30. Cohen JL, Segal KR, Witriol I, et al. Cardiorespiratory responses to ballet exercise and the VO2max of elite ballet dancers. Med Sci Sports Exerc 1982;14(3):212–7.
31. Wyon MA. Testing the aesthetic athlete. In: Winter E, Jones A, Davison R, et al, editors. Sport and exercise physiology testing guidelines: British Association of Sport and Exercise Science testing guidelines, vol. 2. Abingdon: Routledge, Taylor and Francis Group; 2007. p. 249–62.
32. Helms ER, Zinn C, Rowlands DS, et al. A systematic review of dietary protein during caloric restriction in resistance trained lean athletes: a case for higher intakes. Int J Sport Nutr Exerc Metab 2014;24(2):127–38.
33. Mettler S, Mitchell N, Tipton KD. Increased protein intake reduces lean body mass loss during weight loss in athletes. Med Sci Sports Exerc 2010;42(2): 326–37.
34. Brown AF, Bach C, Almeida GT de, et al. Body composition and performance capabilities based on protein intake in collegiate dancers: a pilot study. J Sports Sci 2017;5.

35. Constantini NW, Dubnov G, Lebrun CM. The menstrual cycle and sport performance. Clin Sports Med 2005;24(2):e51–82, xiii-xiv.
36. Oosthuyse T, Bosch AN. The effect of the menstrual cycle on exercise metabolism: implications for exercise performance in eumenorrhoeic women. Sports Med 2010;40(3):207–27.
37. Rickenlund A, Eriksson MJ, Schenck-Gustafsson K, et al. Amenorrhea in female athletes is associated with endothelial dysfunction and unfavorable lipid profile. J Clin Endocrinol Metab 2005;90(3):1354–9.
38. Fosnacht K, Calderone SM. Undergraduate financial stress, financial self- efficacy, and major choice: A multi-institutional study. J Financ Ther 2017;8(1): 107–23.

Special Considerations for Growing Dancers

Bridget J. Quinn, MD*, Charles Scott, MD, Andrea Stracciolini, MD

KEYWORDS

- Sports/dance specialization • Sleep • Mental health • Growth
- Musculoskeletal imbalances • Energy availability • Bone health

KEY POINTS

- Sleep duration and quality is an important component of health maintenance in young dancers.
- The adolescent growth spurt increases the dancers' risk for injury.
- Adolescent dancers are at increased risk of mental health problems caused by a variety of psychosocial stressors, including perfectionism and burnout.
- There is a high prevalence of disordered eating/eating disorders in dancers.[1] Improper nutrition and suboptimal energy intake can have negative metabolic and musculoskeletal health effects (both short and long term) that result in increased risk for injury and decrease training/performance capability.

ANDREA STRACCIOLINI, MD
Dance Specialization Epidemiology

Sleep duration and quality is an important component of the health maintenance of all young dancers. The interplay between dance specialization, dance training hours and participation, and sleep duration has not been extensively investigated in young dancers. Sport specialization occurs when young athletes focus on 1 sport, possibly at the exclusion of all others, and typically results in year-round participation and high-intensity training in a single sport. Specialized young athletes, including gymnasts, figure skaters, and divers, are more likely to train at greater volumes,[1] and maintain a higher risk for overuse injury.[2] Under this umbrella, young dancers maintain similar patterns of participation and risk for injury. In a recent longitudinal questionnaire study of ballet dancers, 79% solely participated in dance, 51% of dancers quit other sports to focus on dance, and 98% participated in dance more than 8 months in the year. Furthermore, 43% of the dancer cohort were categorized as specialized, and more than one-third of specialized dancers reported not fully participating in dance because

Division of Sports Medicine, Department of Orthopedic Surgery, Boston Children's Hospital, 319 Longwood Avenue, Boston, MA 02115, USA
* Corresponding author.
E-mail address: Bridget.Quinn@childrens.harvard.edu

Phys Med Rehabil Clin N Am 32 (2021) 75–86
https://doi.org/10.1016/j.pmr.2020.09.005
1047-9651/21/© 2020 Elsevier Inc. All rights reserved.

pmr.theclinics.com

of injury/illness compared with 14% of dancers characterized as nonspecialized dancers ($P = .060$).[3]

Sleep and Specialization in Dance

The increased demand and volume of dance training as children progress through puberty may displace critical sleep hours, indirectly increasing risk for stress and anxiety as well as dance-related injury. Dance training, rehearsal, and performance schedules, including both time and volume, are a pertinent factor that may directly affect sleep duration.

As young dancers continue to participate at increasing competitive levels while specializing early, training volume inherently increases.[1] The increase in training volume that is inherent to specialization may directly affect physical and psychological health by altering sleep duration and quality. Training schedules, including both time and volume in athletes, is a pertinent factor that may directly affect sleep duration. To this point, studies have shown that early morning starts reduce sleep duration and increase pretraining fatigue levels.[4,5] Recent studies have shown a relationship between training load and sleep in youth athletes, reporting the negative impact of training load on well-being exacerbated by reduced sleep, and minimized by increased sleep.[6]

The adverse effects of short sleep duration on injury are just now beginning to be realized in the literature. The literature supports the link between sports injury and sleep duration.[7] Adolescent athletes who sleep less than 8 hours per night on average are almost twice as likely to sustain a sport-related injury.[8] Luke and colleagues[9] reported that, among athletes 6 to 18 years old, there was an association between physician-determined fatigue-related sports injuries and sleeping less than or equal to 6 hours the night before the injury ($P = .028$). These findings continue to support a possible link between sports-related injury and sleep habits among athletes. Although no studies to date have investigated these links in dancers uniquely, the data can be extrapolated to include young dancers in order to encourage continued guidance surrounding sleep duration and quality surrounding dance training, performances, and competitions.

Sleep Recommendations and Mental Health in Dancers

The current age-based sleep recommendations for children from the American Academy of Pediatrics (AAP) (2016)[10] and the American Academy of Sleep Medicine (2016)[11] state that children 6 to 12 years old should get 9 to 12 hours of sleep per night, adolescents 13 to 18 years old 8 to 10 hours of sleep per night, and adults 19 years of age and older should receive at least 7 hours of sleep per night. The importance of sleep in children, and the relationship to mental and physical health, may be underrecognized when caring for young dancers. In a recent study (Stracciolini and colleagues, unpublished data), roughly 40% of athletes, including dancers, failed to meet the current sleep recommendations, and, when accounting for age, almost half of all adolescents in the range of 13 to 18 years of age did not meet current sleep recommendations. For comparison, Patte and colleagues[12] similarly reported on sleep trajectories in Canadian youth and found that less than half of youth reported meeting the sleep guideline of 8 to 10 hours per night, with boys more likely to report longer sleep duration compared with girls. Chaput and Janssen[13] reported that nearly one-third of Canadian youth failed to meet the current sleep recommendations, with nominal differences between the girls and boys.

Sleep and mental health have been linked in population-based studies.[14–18] In college students, short sleep duration and daytime sleepiness have been shown to have a direct association with an increased risk for mental disorder.[16] Among high school students, shorter sleep duration during school nights is associated with daytime sleepiness and depression symptoms.[19] Young dancers pose unique concerns surrounding sleep associations with regard to health and well-being. The physical and emotional demands of dance participation may contribute both positively and negatively to sleep quality and quantity. On the positive side, it has been well established that increased physical activity for children and adolescents improves sleep quality.[20] In addition, physical activity decreases stress and anxiety, and improves mental health, further increasing the likelihood of improved sleep hygiene and overall quality of life.

Questionnaire data on sleep habits and mental health in a cohort of dancers 12 to 17 years of age found the mean hours of sleep per night to be 7.8 ± 0.9 hours, and greater than 50% of the dancers reported less than 8 hours of sleep per night. As expected, sleep hours per night decreased with age. Interestingly, the mean total screen time for dancers was 3.4 ± 2.1 h/d, and 12% of the dancer cohort reported a history of anxiety.[21] Although this research cannot establish cause and effect, anticipatory guidance when caring for young dancers surrounding the importance of sleep quantity and quality should be a priority in order to support both mental and physical health.

STRENGTH AND FLEXIBILITY IMBALANCE AS RISK FACTOR FOR INJURY
Charles Scott, MD

The adolescent growth spurt generally occurs between the ages of 11 and 14 years in girls and 13 to 21 in boys and is associated with increased vulnerability to injury in dancers. Risk factors for injury in this group include extrinsic factors, such as training environment (eg, footwear, dance surface), volume, intensity, and quality.[22,23] Intrinsic factors in adolescent dancers include imbalances in strength and flexibility resulting from rapid physical growth. Intrinsic and extrinsic factors work synergistically and are associated with increased injury incidence.[22,24] During periods of rapid growth, longitudinal skeletal elongation occurs first, with the soft tissues, including ligaments and tendons, elongating secondarily in response to bone growth.[25,26] The result of this type of imbalance is a relative loss of flexibility and increased tension around the joints of the lumbar spine, pelvis, and lower extremities. This environment of imbalance and tension poses significant injury risk for young dancers. In a cross-sectional cohort study of 1336 nonprofessional female dancers aged 8 to 16 years, a higher rate of injury in older dancers was associated with this increased rate of bone growth relative to the ligaments and tendons.[27] In addition, the growth period has been associated with relative muscle strength decrement resulting in decreased coordination and neuromuscular control.[24]

The impact of growth-associated strength and flexibility imbalances is well shown in 2 of the most common overuse injuries seen in young dancers: pelvic apophysitis and lumbar spondylolysis. Apophysitis refers to an inflammatory response to repetitive traction stress at a secondary ossification center in a skeletally immature patient. A cross-sectional epidemiologic study of 181 injured dancers aged 5 to 16 years found that apophysitis accounted for 6.3% of reported injuries.[28] In Irish step dancers, the rate of apophyseal injuries is even higher (11.4%).[29] In pediatric sports, tibial tuberosity apophysitis (Osgood-Schlatter disease) and os calcis apophysitis (Sever disease) are common, occurring largely in running and jumping athletes. In young dancers, pelvic apophysitis, and particularly anterior iliac crest apophysitis, is more common. The anterior ilium corresponds to the origin of the external oblique, transversus abdominis, and tensor fascia lata muscles and, in dance, is subject to considerable repetitive stress as a result of serial ballistic hip flexion and abduction movements. These stresses are increased in the setting of tight and weak hip external rotators and abductors,[28] creating a perfect environment for the development of apophyseal injury.

Growth-related biomechanical imbalances can also affect the alignment and function of the lumbar spine, as can be seen in lumbar spondylolysis. Pars interarticularis stress injuries are a common cause of low back pain and dysfunction in young dancers.[23,30] In a cross-sectional epidemiologic study of 178 dancers aged 5 to 17 years, lumbar spondylolysis accounted for 4.5% of all reported dance injuries.[30] Although epidemiologic data in dancers are limited, prevalence would be expected to exceed that of a general pediatric population. In a prospective study of 153 pediatric patients (<19 years old) with back pain of more than 2 weeks' duration, the prevalence of lumbar spondylolysis was 39.7%.[31] Biomechanically, a combination of muscle weakness/tightness and poor anatomic alignment frequently manifests as lumbar lordosis, an important risk factor for spondylolysis.[23] During the adolescent growth spurt, weakening of the core musculature accompanied by tightening of the lumbodorsal fascia, hamstrings, and anterior hip musculature predispose to lumbar lordosis. The effect is often compounded by training errors that encourage dancers to increase hip external rotation through a combination of anterior pelvic tilt and swaying of the lumbar spine.[23] Treatment of spondylolysis typically requires a prolonged period of complete rest from sports-related activity and focused rehabilitation to address and correct underlying strength, flexibility, and technical deficits.[32]

Iliac crest apophysitis and lumbar spondylolysis are 2 examples of a wide variety of overuse injuries seen in growing dancers. Treatments for these injuries can significantly interfere with young dancers' training programs and performance at a pivotal time in their careers.[33] A preventive approach is recommended to address underlying technical and biomechanical imbalances before the growth spurt and to equip dancers with knowledge and skills to address deficits even before injury occurs.[25,29,30] Individualized conditioning programs based on injury history and functional movement screening have been shown to prevent dance injury.[34] As in baseball, where mandated pitch counts and rest periods have helped prevent pitching-related injury,[35] careful attention to volume and periodization of dance training even before the adolescent growth spurt may help prevent injury while improving dancers' performance readiness.[36] Additional research is needed to help guide the development of specific prevention and treatment recommendations.

MENTAL HEALTH CONSIDERATIONS
Charles Scott, MD

Adolescent dancers are at increased risk of mental health problems because of a variety of psychosocial stressors. Some aspects of mental health distress among young dancers intersect with those of a general population of young athletes, whereas other aspects are more specific to the unique training and performance demands placed on young dancers. Like young athletes, dancers are increasingly subject to early specialization and high performance demands.[37] Challenging daily schedules, often with condensed academic and social time to allow for intensive training, can result in social isolation, altered family relationships, overdependence on others, and loss of a sense of control.[38,39] Adolescent dancers may be particularly prone to perfectionism, problems involving body image, and burnout.[40]

PERFECTIONISM IN DANCERS

A growing body of literature points to the central role of perfectionism as an underlying maladaptive personality feature seen in many young dancers that can predispose to psychological and physical distress. Perfectionism is a multidimensional trait characterized by high, often unattainable, personal standards and compulsive self-evaluative behaviors.[41] This trait can be difficult to distinguish from adaptive achievement striving.[40,42,43] With perfectionism, the sense of self-worth becomes dependent on the perceived appreciation of others and the ability to do things right.[40] The dance training environment may contribute to this effect. Mainwaring and Finney[44] proposed that young dancers are trained to hold perfectionistic beliefs and values through a formalized system of harsh criticism from instructors, reinforced by their peers and parents, in such a way as to instill unattainable standards and rigid self-scrutiny. Perfectionism can also influence dancers' perceptions of their physical appearance, leading to body objectification and dysmorphia.[42,45] A direct correlation has been established between perfectionism and the development of eating disorders in young dancers.[43,45]

The implications of perfectionism in the athletic and performing arts communities have been widely discussed in the literature, whereas little has been written about its management. Early approaches to management of perfectionism were limited in their effect and focused on developing learning environments where dancers could learn self-efficacy and autonomy while feeling valued by teachers and peers.[43,46] Reports of early therapeutic approaches suggested a high level of treatment resistance, although cognitive behavior therapy has more recently shown promise in addressing distorted thinking and dysfunctional behaviors that accompany perfectionism.[43]

BURNOUT IN DANCERS

There is a close relationship between perfectionism and burnout in young dancers. In a recent survey of 91 student and professional ballet dancers (mean age, 17.23 years), those with perfectionism traits reported more frequent burnout symptoms (reduced sense of accomplishment, physical and emotional exhaustion, and dance devaluation) than those reporting nonperfectionism.[41] Factors contributing to burnout include high training volume and intensive time commitment at the expense of other activities (eg, academics, family time), demanding expectations (from self, teachers, parents), decreased sense of personal control, and negative feedback.[47] Although conceptually, burnout may seem counterintuitive in settings where personal commitment and striving are high, such as in athletics or the performing arts, burnout may be the result of people caring too much about their work.[48] Burnout has been shown to have important consequences for performance and well-being. In young athletes, dropping out as a result of burnout is associated with increased risk for obesity, depression, and reduced academic performance.[49] Although no formal recommendations exist to guide burnout prevention in dancers, the AAP and the American Medical Society for Sports Medicine (AMSSM) have published guidelines for the prevention of burnout in athletes, which may be extrapolated to burnout management in dancers.[39,50] These recommendations include emphasizing skill development more than competition, keeping training fun, regularly scheduled time away from sport (weekly and annually), and focusing on wellness preparing individuals to recognize training stress.[50] Additional research into the effects of interventions addressing perfectionism and burnout will help guide formal recommendations for young dancers.

RELATIVE ENERGY DEFICIENCY IN DANCERS
Bridget J. Quinn, MD

Dance as an aesthetic art form places dancers at all skill levels at increased risk for disordered thoughts and behaviors in an effort to achieve the supposedly ideal body type.[51] Disordered eating often develops during adolescence, when dancers enter puberty with its associated body changes, and increase their commitment to the art form.[52] There is a high prevalence of disordered eating/eating disorders in dancers.[51] Improper nutrition and suboptimal energy intake can have negative metabolic and musculoskeletal health effects (both short and long term) and result in increased risk for injury and decrease training/performance capability. It is imperative that clinicians be aware of the importance of nutrition, energy availability (EA), signs/symptoms of underfueling, and diagnosis and treatment in dancer athletes.

There is a spectrum of risk factors that contribute to dancers developing low EA with or without disordered thoughts and behaviors. Young dancers have significant demands on their time, including school, dance, and friend/family commitments. Young dancers may inadvertently be in a low-energy state because of lack of understanding of what their body needs and/or lack of time and resources to prepare and consume food. The term relative energy deficiency in sport (RED-S) was coined in 2014 by the International Olympic Committee.[53] It is an evolution of the female athlete triad's 3 interrelated conditions of suboptimal EA, menstrual dysfunction, and low bone density. The RED-S model expands the core concept of suboptimal EA to include both women and men and the multiple body systems affected by reduced EA. All athletes are at risk for RED-S, but there are certain lean-type sports that are at higher risk, such as dance.[54]

There are various ways to evaluate whether a dancer is in a relative energy-deficient state. An athlete's EA is calculated by subtracting the energy expended during exercise (energy expended during exercise in excess of energy needed for normal physiologic function) from the energy intake, normalized to the fat-free mass (FFM) (kcal/kg FFM/d).[55] When an athlete's EA is less than 30 kcal/kg FFM/d, the dancer may start to experience negative metabolic and endocrine effects of being in a reduced-energy state.[55] However, 30 kcal/kg should not be used as an absolute EA threshold, because individuals have shown hormonal and performance disturbances at more than 30 kcal/kg/d, with some studies suggesting an EA of at least 45 kcal/kg FFM/d for optimal functioning, particularly in growing athletes.[55,56] In assessing a dancer's nutritional needs, there are various factors to take into account, including resting metabolic rate (RMR), energy output beyond RMR, dietary sensitivities, allergies, and preferences. It is recommended to coordinate care in assessing a young dancer's energy needs with a registered sports dietitian who also works with a pediatric/adolescent population.

When the human body perceives itself to be in a low-energy state, it enters a conservation mode and shunts energy away from reproduction and growth.[2] In females with suboptimal EA, this can be marked by a variety of menstrual disturbances. Dancers, in particular those with lower body mass index (BMI), may experience a delay in onset of their menstrual cycle (menarche).[57,58] Dancers who have had more years of dance starting at a younger age are more likely to have a delayed onset of menarche.[59] Primary amenorrhea is defined by the absence of a menstrual cycle by the age of 15 years in the setting of normal growth and development of secondary sexual characteristics.[60] Once a young woman starts getting her menstrual cycle, it can be irregular for 1 to 2 years. A normal menstrual cycle is every 28 days, plus or minus 7 days. Adolescent menstrual cycles can range from every 21 to 45 days.[61] Dancers with suboptimal EA may experience increased time intervals between cycles, skipped cycles, or go prolonged periods of time without a menstrual cycle. Oligomenorrhea is defined as infrequent menstruation, with cycles at intervals greater than or equal to 45 days.[61] Secondary amenorrhea is defined as missed regular menses for greater than or equal to 3 months consecutively or absence of irregular menses for greater than or equal to 6 months.[62] Dancers who experience increased levels of psychogenic stress, suboptimal EA and nutrition, weight fluctuations, low percentage body fat, and high levels of exercise are at risk for functional hypothalamic amenorrhea, resulting from abnormal signaling through the hypothalamic-pituitary-gonadal axis.[53,60]

Male athletes in certain lean-type sports are also at increased risk for low EA and its associated endocrine and metabolic effects,[53,63,64] including an associated negative impact on reproductive health, such as testosterone levels and bone health. Males may need to be in a more significant low-energy state to see these negative effects, but this area of RED-S research is expanding.[14] A low RMR ratio (RMR_R) has been used as a surrogate marker for low EA.[65] The RMR represents the body's energy needs for physiologic functioning (circulation, breathing, thermoregulation, and so forth) at rest. A low ratio between the measured RMR ($_MRMR$) and the predicted RMR ($_PRMR$) has been reported in dancers with low EA and amenorrhea. In Staal and colleagues'[65] study using a low RMR_R as a marker of low EA, the $_MRMR$ was measured via a ventilation hood system. The $_PRMR$ was measured via the Cunningham equation, Harris-Benedict equation, and different tissue compartments from the whole-body dual energy x-ray absorptiometry (DXA) assessment. A RMR_R of less than 0.9 represented suppressed RMR. In male dancers, a low RMR_R was associated with high training volumes. The prevalence of low EA in male dancers and its associated metabolic and endocrine effects has not been fully elucidated. However, there is growing research in the metabolic health of exercising male athletes.

Bone health has contributions from both the environment, including nutrition and physical activity, and genetics.[66,67] Low EA is associated with negative effects on bone health. Adolescence is a critical time for bone mass accrual. Approximately 90% of a woman's bone mass is built by the age of 18 to 19 years.[68,69] Insults such as improper nutrition and suboptimal EA can result in irreversible effects on dancers' short-term and long-term bone health.[59] However, the prevalence of low bone mineral density in female dancers is not fully understood.[70] Some studies suggest that dancers have higher bone densities because of their dance training, whereas others report an increased risk of low bone density.[16] The research to date is suboptimal in assessing bone health in dancers. The nondancer female athlete population has been more extensively researched and shows a negative correlation between low EA and peak bone mass development and bone health.[71–75] Further high-quality research is needed regarding bone health in dancers, in particular dancers with low EA.

It is important for practitioners to have RED-S on their differential when evaluating a dancer. Markers of low EA/RED-S include, but are not limited to, bony stress injuries, recurrent injuries, delayed injury healing, a decrease in weight on the dancer's growth chart, low BMI, delayed menarche, menstrual dysfunction, altered mood, performance decline, and fatigue.[12] These markers can be related to issues outside of low EA/RED-S, so the practitioner should acknowledge the at-risk dancer and exclude potential secondary causes. The initial evaluation includes blood work to assess for immunosuppression as marked by leukopenia, anemia, decrease in iron storage via ferritin levels, comprehensive metabolic panel to assess electrolytes, kidney function, minerals, including calcium, magnesium, and phosphorous, and 25-hydroxy vitamin D. Thyroid dysfunction can be a source of altered menstruation or a marker of low

EA, with a low liothyronine level being associated with low EA.[76] A hormonal panel including estradiol, follicle-stimulating hormone, luteinizing hormone, thyroid-stimulating hormone, free T4 (thyroxine), and prolactin should be assessed in those dancers with amenorrhea, with polycystic ovary syndrome screening as well, in the correct clinical scenario.[77] DXA can be obtained using Z-scores (comparison with age-appropriate norms) to evaluate the dancer's bone density. In children and adolescents, preferred scan locations are the lumbar spine and total body less head. The whole-body scan can also provide measurements of body composition, with percent body fat Z-scores helpful in guiding weight goals for menstrual resumption. Treatment is designed to address the underlying issue of low EA, with the eventual result of spontaneous regular menses in female dancers. It is not recommended to start amenorrheic or oligomenorrheic dancers on exogenous hormones such as oral contraceptive pills, because these mask the underlying issue. However, in the process of treatment, if resumption of menses has not occurred with 6 months of nutritional, psychological, and/or exercise modification interventions, transdermal estrogen with cyclic oral progesterone is recommended to help enhance bone mineral density.[77] Treatment requires an interdisciplinary approach, including the medical sports physician/primary care doctor, skilled sports dietitian familiar with the dancer athlete, and sports psychologist. The ability for the dancer to continue to train and perform depends on the dancer's medical status and is ultimately a team-based decision.

The dancer as an aesthetic athlete is at risk for low EA and its associated negative metabolic and training/performance effects. Although further research is needed, in particular in the realm of bone health and male athletes, the data thus far support screening and intervening with an interdisciplinary team to help support the short-term and long-term health of the dancers.

CLINICS CARE POINTS

- Dancer sleep duration and quality should be part of their clinical evaluation.
- Consider training modifications during the adolescent growth spurt.
- Cognitive behavioral therapy is a potentially useful tool for dancers with perfectionism.
- Screening and early intervention of dancers with low energy availability can contribute positively to short and long term health.

DISCLOSURE

The authors have nothing to disclose.

REFERENCES

1. Field AE, Tepolt FA, Yang DS, et al. Injury Risk Associated With Sports Specialization and Activity Volume in Youth. Orthop J Sports Med 2019;7(9). 2325967119870124.

2. Bell DR, Post EG, Biese K, et al. Sport Specialization and Risk of Overuse Injuries: A Systematic Review With Meta-analysis. Pediatrics 2018;142(3):e20180657.

3. Stracciolini A, GM, Sugimoto D, et al. Early Sport Specialization in Dance. American Medical Society for Sports Medicine (AMSSM). J Oral Poster Presentation. Houston, April 12-17, 2019.

4. Sargent C, Lastella M, Halson SL, et al. The impact of training schedules on the sleep and fatigue of elite athletes. Chronobiol Int 2014;31(10):1160–8.

5. Sargent C, Halson S, Roach GD. Sleep or swim? Early-morning training severely restricts the amount of sleep obtained by elite swimmers. Eur J Sport Sci 2014; 14(Suppl 1):S310–5.

6. Watson A, Brickson S. Impaired Sleep Mediates the Negative Effects of Training Load on Subjective Well-Being in Female Youth Athletes. Sports Health 2018; 10(3):244–9.

7. Gao B, Dwivedi S, Milewski MD, et al. Lack of Sleep and Sports Injuries in Adolescents: A Systematic Review and Meta-analysis. J Pediatr Orthop 2019;39(5): e324–33.

8. Milewski MD, Skaggs DL, Bishop GA, et al. Chronic lack of sleep is associated with increased sports injuries in adolescent athletes. J Pediatr orthopedics 2014;34(2):129–33.

9. Luke A, Lazaro RM, Bergeron MF, et al. Sports-related injuries in youth athletes: is overscheduling a risk factor? Clin J Sport Med 2011;21(4):307–14.

10. Paruthi S, Brooks LJ, D'Ambrosio C, et al. Consensus Statement of the American Academy of Sleep Medicine on the Recommended Amount of Sleep for Healthy Children: Methodology and Discussion. J Clin Sleep Med 2016;12(11):1549–61.

11. Lewin DS, Wolfson AR, Bixler EO, et al. Duration Isn't Everything. Healthy Sleep in Children and Teens: Duration, Individual Need and Timing. J Clin Sleep Med 2016;12(11):1439–41.

12. Patte KA, Cole AG, Qian W, et al. Youth sleep durations and school start times: a cross-sectional analysis of the COMPASS study. Sleep Health 2017;3(6):432–6.

13. Chaput JP, Janssen I. Sleep duration estimates of Canadian children and adolescents. J Sleep Res 2016;25(5):541–8.

14. Castro LS, Castro J, Hoexter MQ, et al. Depressive symptoms and sleep: a population-based polysomnographic study. Psychiatry Res 2013;210(3):906–12.

15. Wilsmore BR, Grunstein RR, Fransen M, et al. Sleep habits, insomnia, and daytime sleepiness in a large and healthy community-based sample of New Zealanders. J Clin Sleep Med 2013;9(6):559–66.

16. Dickinson DL, Wolkow AP, Rajaratnam SMW, et al. Personal sleep debt and daytime sleepiness mediate the relationship between sleep and mental health outcomes in young adults. Depress Anxiety 2018;35(8):775–83.

17. Forbes EE, Bertocci MA, Gregory AM, et al. Objective sleep in pediatric anxiety disorders and major depressive disorder. J Am Acad Child Adolesc Psychiatry 2008;47(2):148–55.

18. Joao K, Jesus SN, Carmo C, et al. The impact of sleep quality on the mental health of a non-clinical population. Sleep Med 2018;46:69–73.

19. O'Brien EM, Mindell JA. Sleep and risk-taking behavior in adolescents. Behav Sleep Med 2005;3(3):113–33.

20. Miller MA, Kruisbrink M, Wallace J, et al. Sleep duration and incidence of obesity in infants, children, and adolescents: a systematic review and meta-analysis of prospective studies. Sleep 2018;41(4):1–19.

21. Stracciolini A, Stein CJ, Kinney S, et al. Associations Between Sedentary Behaviors, Sleep Patterns, and BMI in Young Dancers Attending a Summer Intensive Dance Training Program. J Dance Med Sci 2017;21(3):102–8.

22. Bowerman EA, Whatman C, Harris N, et al. A Review of the Risk Factors for Lower Extremity Overuse Injuries in Young Elite Female Ballet Dancers. J Dance Med Sci 2015;19(2):51–6.

23. Micheli L. Back Pain in Dancers. Clin Sports Med 1983;2:473–84.

24. Poggini L, Losasso S, Iannone S. Injuries during the Dancer's growth spurt. J Dance Med Sci 1999;3(2):73–9.

25. Micheli L. Injuries in Growing Athletes. Orthop Clin North Am 1983;14:337–59.
26. Steinberg N, Siev-Ner I, Peleg S, et al. Injury patterns in young, non-professional dancers. J Sports Sci 2011;29(1):47–54.
27. Steinberg N, Siev-Ner I. Injuries in Female Dancers Aged 8 to 16 Years. J Athl Train 2013;48(1):118–22.
28. Yin AX, Geminiani E, Quinn B, et al. The Evaluation of Strength, Flexibility, and Functional Performance in the Adolescent Ballet Dancer During Intensive Dance Training. PM R 2019;11(7):722–30.
29. Stein CJ, Tyson KD, Johnson VM, et al. Injuries in Irish Dance. J Dance Med Sci 2013;17(4):159–64.
30. Yin AX, Sugimoto D, Martin DJ, et al. Pediatric Dance Injuries: A Cross-Sectional Epidemiological Study. PM R 2016;8(4):348–55.
31. Nitta A, Sakai T, Goda Y, et al. Prevalence of Symptomatic Lumbar Spondylolysis in Pediatric Patients. Orthopedics 2016;39(3):e434–7.
32. Goetzinger S, Courtney S, Yee K, et al. Spondylolysis in Young Athletes: An Overview Emphasizing Nonoperative Management. J Sports Med 2020;2020:1–15.
33. Frush TJ, Lindenfeld TN. Peri-epiphyseal and Overuse Injuries in Adolescent Athletes. Sports Health 2009;1(3):201–11.
34. Allen M, Nevill HM, Brooks A, et al. The Effect of a Comprehensive Injury Audit Program on Injury Incidence in Ballet: A 3-Year Prospective Study. Clin J Sport Med 2013;23(5):373–8.
35. Bakshi NK, Inclan PM, Kirsch JM, et al. Current Workload Recommendations in Baseball Pitchers: A Systematic Review. Am J Sports Med 2020;48(1):229–41.
36. Wyon M. Preparing to Perform. J Dance Med Sci 2010;14(2):67–72.
37. Stracciolini A, Sugimoto D, Quinn B. Early Sport Specialization in Dance. Oral Poster Presentation presented at the: American Medical Society for Sports Medicine (AMSSM). Houston, April 12-17, 2019.
38. Grove JR, Main LC, Sharp L. Stressors, Recovery Processes, and Manifestations of Training Distress in Dance. J Dance Med Sci 2013;17(2):70–8.
39. Brenner JS, Council on Sports Medicine and Fitness. Sports Specialization and Intensive Training in Young Athletes. Pediatrics 2016;138(3):e20162148.
40. van Staden A, Myburgh CPH, Poggenpoel M. A Psycho-Education Model to Enhance the Self-Development and Mental Health of Classical Dancers. J Dance Med Sci 2009;13(1):20–8.
41. Nordin-Bates SM, Raedeke TD, Madigan DJ. Perfectionism, Burnout, and Motivation in Dance. J Dance Med Sci 2017;21(3):115–22.
42. Cumming J, Duda JL. Profiles of perfectionism, body-related concerns, and indicators of psychological health in vocational dance students: An investigation of the 2 × 2 model of perfectionism. Psychol Sport Exerc 2012;13(6):729–38.
43. Hall HK, Hill AP. Perfectionism, dysfunctional achievement striving and burnout in aspiring athletes: the motivational implications for performing artists. Theatre, Dance & Performance Training 2012;3(2):216–28.
44. Mainwaring LM, Finney C. Psychological Risk Factors and Outcomes of Dance Injury: A Systematic Review. J Dance Med Sci 2017;21(3):87–96.
45. Anshel M. Sources of Disordered Eating Patterns Between Ballet Dancers and Non-dancers. J Sport Behav 2004;27(2):115–33.
46. Buckroyd J. The Student Dancer: Emotional Aspects of the Teaching and Learning of Dance. Dance Res J 2001;33(1):109–12.
47. Brenner JS, LaBotz M, Sugimoto D, et al. The Psychosocial Implications of Sport Specialization in Pediatric Athletes. J Athl Train 2019;54(10):1021–9.

48. Goodger KI, Jones MI. Burnout: a darker side to performance. Oxford University Press; 2012. https://doi.org/10.1093/oxfordhb/9780199731763.013.0030.
49. Cresswell S, Eklund RC. Athlete Burnout: Conceptual Confusion, Current Research and Future Research Directions. In: Hanton S, Mellalieu SD, editors. Literature Reviews in Sport Psychology. Nova Science Publishers; 2006. p. 91–126.
50. DiFiori JP, Benjamin HJ, Brenner JS, et al. Overuse injuries and burnout in youth sports: a position statement from the American Medical Society for Sports Medicine. Br J Sports Med 2014;48(4):287–8.
51. Hincapié CA, Cassidy JD. Disordered Eating, Menstrual Disturbances, and Low Bone Mineral Density in Dancers: A Systematic Review. Arch Phys Med Rehabil 2010;91(11):1777–89.e1.
52. Smolak L, Murnen SK, Ruble AE. Female athletes and eating problems: A meta-analysis. Int J Eat Disord 2000;27(4):371–80.
53. Mountjoy M, Sundgot-Borgen J, Burke L, et al. The IOC consensus statement: beyond the Female Athlete Triad—Relative Energy Deficiency in Sport (RED-S). Br J Sports Med 2014;48(7):491–7.
54. Thompson RA, Sherman RT. Eating disorders in sport. New York: Routledge; 2011.
55. Loucks AB, Kiens B, Wright HH. Energy availability in athletes. J Sports Sci 2011; 29(Suppl 1):S7–15.
56. Melin AK, Heikura IA, Tenforde A, et al. Energy Availability in Athletics: Health, Performance, and Physique. Int J Sport Nutr Exerc Metab 2019;29(2):152–64.
57. Stracciolini A, Quinn BJ, Geminiani F, et al. Body Mass Index and Menstrual Patterns in Dancers. Clin Pediatr (Phila) 2017;56(1):49–54.
58. Burckhardt P, Wynn E, Krieg M-A, et al. The Effects of Nutrition, Puberty and Dancing on Bone Density in Adolescent Ballet Dancers. J Dance Med Sci 2011;15(2):51–60.
59. Valentino R, Savastano S, Tommaselli AP, et al. The Influence of Intense Ballet Training on Trabecular Bone Mass, Hormone Status, and Gonadotropin Structure in Young Women. The Journal of Clinical Endocrinology and Metabolism 2001; 86(10):4674–8.
60. Practice Committee of American Society for Reproductive Medicine. Current evaluation of amenorrhea. Fertil Sterility 2008;90(5):S219–25.
61. ACOG Committee on Adolescent Health Care. ACOG Committee Opinion No. 349, November 2006: Menstruation in girls and adolescents: using the menstrual cycle as a vital sign. Obstet Gynecol 2006;108(5):1323–8.
62. Klein DA, Poth MA. Amenorrhea: an approach to diagnosis and management. Am Fam Physician 2013;87(11):781–8.
63. Mountjoy M, Sundgot-Borgen JK, Burke LM, et al. IOC consensus statement on relative energy deficiency in sport (RED-S): 2018 update. Br J Sports Med 2018;52(11):687–97.
64. Hackney AC. Hypogonadism in Exercising Males: Dysfunction or Adaptive-Regulatory Adjustment? Front Endocrinol (Lausanne) 2020;11. https://doi.org/10.3389/fendo.2020.00011.
65. Staal S, Sjödin A, Fahrenholtz I, et al. Low RMR ratio as a Surrogate Marker for Energy Deficiency, the Choice of Predictive Equation Vital for Correctly Identifying Male and Female Ballet Dancers at Risk. Int J Sport Nutr Exerc Metab 2018;28(4):412–8.
66. Krall EA, Dawson-Hughes B. Heritable and life-style determinants of bone mineral density. J Bone Miner Res 1993;8(1):1–9.

67. Naganathan V, Macgregor A, Snieder H, et al. Gender Differences in the Genetic Factors Responsible for Variation in Bone Density and Ultrasound. J Bone Miner Res 2002;17(4):725–33.
68. Bailey DA, Mckay HA, Mirwald RL, et al. A Six-Year Longitudinal Study of the Relationship of Physical Activity to Bone Mineral Accrual in Growing Children: The University of Saskatchewan Bone Mineral Accrual Study. J Bone Miner Res 1999;14(10):1672–9.
69. Baxter-Jones AD, Faulkner RA, Forwood MR, et al. Bone mineral accrual from 8 to 30 years of age: An estimation of peak bone mass. J Bone Miner Res 2011;26(8): 1729–39.
70. Amorim T, Wyon M, Maia J, et al. Prevalence of Low Bone Mineral Density in Female Dancers. Sports Med 2015;45(2):257–68.
71. Papageorgiou M, Dolan E, Elliott-Sale KJ, et al. Reduced energy availability: implications for bone health in physically active populations. Eur J Nutr 2018;57(3): 847–59.
72. Nattiv A, Loucks AB, Manore MM, et al. American College of Sports Medicine position stand. The female athlete triad. Med Sci Sports Exerc 2007;39(10): 1867–82.
73. Ackerman KE, Nazem T, Chapko D, et al. Bone microarchitecture is impaired in adolescent amenorrheic athletes compared with eumenorrheic athletes and nonathletic controls. J Clin Endocrinol Metab 2011;96(10):3123–33.
74. Ackerman KE, Putman M, Guereca G, et al. Cortical microstructure and estimated bone strength in young amenorrheic athletes, eumenorrheic athletes and non-athletes. Bone 2012;51(4):680–7.
75. De Souza MJ, West SL, Jamal SA, et al. The presence of both an energy deficiency and estrogen deficiency exacerbate alterations of bone metabolism in exercising women. Bone 2008;43(1):140–8.
76. Elliott-Sale KJ, Tenforde AS, Parziale AL, et al. Endocrine Effects of Relative Energy Deficiency in Sport. Int J Sport Nutr Exerc Metab 2018;28(4):335–49.
77. Gordon CM, Ackerman KE, Berga SL, et al. Functional Hypothalamic Amenorrhea: An Endocrine Society Clinical Practice Guideline. J Clin Endocrinol Metab 2017;102(5):1413–39.

Readiness for Dancing En Pointe

Selina Shah, MD

KEYWORDS

- Readiness for pointe • Readiness for dancing en pointe • Pointe readiness
- Dancing en pointe • Advancing to pointe • Ballet pointe • Pointe injuries
- Transition to dancing en pointe

KEY POINTS

- Advancing to pointe requires sufficient maturity, strength, and flexibility and adequate ballet training to develop the necessary skills, including proper technique, alignment, and balance.
- To evaluate if a dancer is ready for pointe requires an understanding of ballet technique.
- This evaluation provides the practitioner and opportunity to evaluate and educate the dancer on 3 key issues: general health, pointe readiness, and technique flaws.

INTRODUCTION

Classical ballet originated in aristocratic Italy in the fifteenth century and has enchanted audiences all around the world since it was popularized under the reign of Louis XIV in France almost 200 years later.[1] Over the centuries, ballet has transformed in terms of its shoes, costumes, and choreography. Dancing *en pointe* (*on the tips of the toes*) was introduced in 1832 by Marie Taglioni at the Paris Opera Ballet, theoretically to allow the audience to see the dancer's feet more clearly.[2] Dancing en pointe became popular quickly and is widely considered a requirement for female dancers to be hired by professional ballet companies. Significantly fewer male dancers also dance en pointe professionally.

For many young ballet dancers, especially female dancers, dancing en pointe is the ultimate goal after years of training, regardless of their future career aspirations. Dancing en pointe is an achievement that requires skill and determination.

Each dance studio has a different method for advancing dancers to pointe work with no standardization; some are stricter than others. For example, some studios may audition each dancer individually, whereas some may advance an entire class without individualizing the decision and others may require an evaluation by a medical professional prior to starting. Unfortunately, in recent years, there has

A Division of BASS Medical Group, 2255 Ygnacio Valley Road, Suite V, Walnut Creek, CA 94598, USA

Phys Med Rehabil Clin N Am 32 (2021) 87–102
https://doi.org/10.1016/j.pmr.2020.09.004
1047-9651/21/© 2020 Elsevier Inc. All rights reserved.

been an increasing trend toward parental pressure influencing advancement of dancers who may not be ready for pointe, which can put a studio in a compromising position in terms of doing what is right while trying to retain students. Some studios maintain strict adherence to the requirements of advancement for pointe work, whereas others may give in to the pressure due to financial burdens for fear of losing students to another studio with less stringent rules. Thus, it is important for health practitioners who may be consulted for recommendations for advancement for pointe work to be comfortable with the evaluation and explain the decision.

Determining if a dancer is ready for pointe requires an understanding of anatomic requirements, ballet technique, and the skills required for pointe work. Ideally, a health practitioner has had danced ballet, either recreationally or professionally, especially dancing en pointe, because this makes evaluating the skill set required for a successful transition to dancing en pointe easier. Even without ballet experience, however, a health practitioner still can perform an evaluation based on understanding how to perform the examination and perhaps gain some practical experience either by taking an introductory ballet class or observing ballet and pointe classes.

BACKGROUND
Ballet Shoes

There are 2 main shoe types in ballet: flexible slippers and pointe shoes. Prior to starting pointe, dancers use flexible slippers (**Fig. 1**) made of either canvas or leather, with a thin outer sole made of leather to allow for turning.

Pointe shoes are complex with detailed anatomy (**Fig. 2**). The shoes are made with a satin fabric that surrounds the foot and a solid toe box with an insole and outer sole. The pointe shoes are tied onto the ankle with a satin or elastic ribbon. The toe box is made of layers of paper, glue, and fabric, usually burlap. The vamp is the top of the toe box that covers the toes. The shank usually is made of shoulder leather and is the supporting spine between the insole and outer sole. The outer sole usually is made of suede to allow for turning when not rising fully to pointe.

Pointe shoes still primarily are handmade, with at least 8 major brands. Each brand manufactures different styles of shoes that vary in the width and shape of the toe box, the length and strength of the shank (double layer for a stronger, more flexible foot), and the length and shape of the vamp. Dancers should take time to be fitted by an experienced pointe shoe fitter given the complexity of the shoe. As dancers age and become more adept at dancing en pointe, dancers should be refit to try other styles or brands of shoes that may be more suitable. More specifically, after dancers are fit for their initial pair, they should be refit each time they need new shoes in the first 6 months to year as they become more comfortable with dancing en pointe. They should be refit every time they change street shoe size or find that the shoes do not feel right subjectively. It is recommended dancers be refit every 1 year to 2 years after they are done growing and if they are recovering from a lower extremity injury. They also should be refit every time they advance a level. Dancers who cannot find a ready-made pointe shoe to fit can order custom-made shoes.

Ideally, dancers should purchase new shoes before they deteriorate structurally (dead shoes), losing the ability to support the foot and ankle. One study showed an increase in midfoot flexion and ankle plantar flexion due to excessive wear.[3] Another study showed increased sway and anterior tibialis activation while en pointe in such shoes.[4] Thus, dancing in dead shoes could lead to an increased risk of injury to the lower extremity.

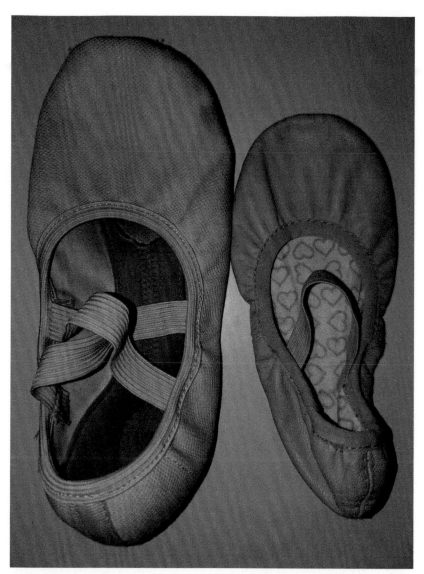

Fig. 1. Flexible ballet slippers. (*Courtesy of* S. Shah, MD, Walnut Creek, CA.)

Ballet Class Structure

Evaluating a dancer for pointe readiness requires an understanding of ballet class structure and technique. Ballet is structured and rigid with minor variations in the 6 major styles taught throughout the world: French, Vaganova (Russian), Cecchetti (Italian), Bournonville (Danish), Royal Ballet (English), and Balanchine (American). Each studio usually teaches ballet and pointe technique based on a single method.

Ballet class begins with *barre*: a warm-up through a series of short, choreographed repetitive movements using the right and left leg for each combination as both the stance leg and then gesture leg. Students hold on to the barre to help them with balance as they warm up by articulating the feet, practicing weight transfers, and

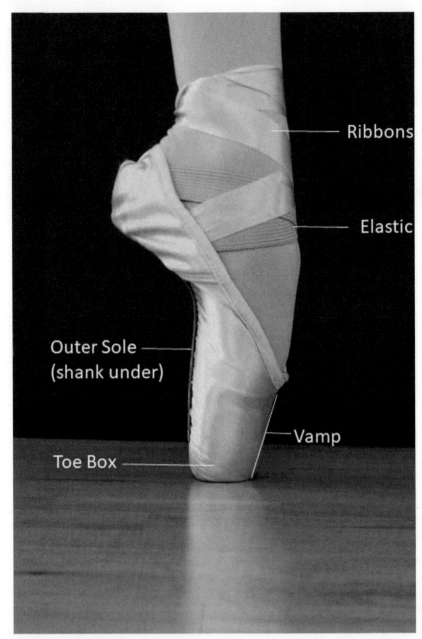

Fig. 2. Pointe shoe anatomy. (*Courtesy of* S. Shah, MD, Walnut Creek, CA.)

activating fine motor muscles, large muscle groups, and the core required of more advanced technique in class. During barre, students start practicing balancing on *relevé* (standing on the metatarsal heads in flat shoes or on the tips of the toes in pointe shoes). After barre, students come to the *center*, where they do a series of combinations in a typical order to work on fast movements, balances on relevé in positions that ideally require some flexibility and strength, and turns. Toward the end of center, the class progresses to jump combinations starting with a series of small jumps, called *petit allegro*. This is followed by *grand allegro*, which is a series of larger jumps. Class ends with *reverence*, where the teacher leads a series of slower movements and end with a courtesy or bow to both the teacher and live musician if present.

In beginning pointe classes, many studios allow dancers to use their pointe shoes at the barre only for the first several months to 1 year and then have the students switch to their regular flexible slippers for the remainder of class. Then, after dancers have developed adequate strength and skill at the barre, they allow the dancers to progress to using their pointe shoes in the center and then the rest of class. Some studios may allow the dancers to use the pointe shoes through the entire class from the beginning, which is more difficult, given that the dancers do not have the support of the barre in the center. It is helpful to know what each studio's philosophy is, because a dancer may be ready for pointe class in a studio that has a more gradual approach to their advancement to pointe work versus a studio who allows the dancer to wear the shoes through the entire class from the beginning.

HEALTH IMPACT
Injuries

Little research exists regarding the physical impact of dancing en pointe. The ability to dance en pointe, however, is an advancement that many strive for and hope to achieve. It is similar to advancing skills in any other athletic endeavor, such as achieving the black belt in tae kwon do or advancing levels in gymnastics. Unfortunately, not all dancers necessarily gain the skills needed to successfully dance en pointe. One case report demonstrated premature growth plate closure of the second metatarsal in dancer who began pointe at the age of 10.[5] The author also has found over the years that most dancers who develop posterior ankle impingement syndrome symptoms either from an os trigonum or Stieda process, do not become symptomatic until they begin dancing en pointe. Another review article found that no evidence exists to demonstrate that dancing en pointe causes hallux valgus deformity. If a dancer is genetically predisposed to developing the deformity, however, excessive pronation may be a contributing factor.[6] One study found that the dancers who spent more the 60 minutes en pointe per week suffered a higher percentage of foot and ankle tendinopathy and back injuries than those who did less than 60 minutes per week.[7] Overall, injury rates in ballet dancers are low. In 1 study of preprofessional full-time ballet dancers, the injury incidence was found to be 2.11 per 1000 hours of dance exposure.[8]

Biomechanics

Dancing en pointe increases overall peak pressure of the total foot by 1.66 times that of dancing barefoot, with the majority of pressure being placed at the hindfoot, followed by the forefoot, followed by the midfoot. The pressure of dancing in pointe shoes in the midfoot is 3.7 times that of dancing barefoot, which may be a contributing factor to metatarsal base stress injuries.[9] Dancing en pointe increases the forces placed on the foot by 12 times the body weight according to another study.[10] Additionally, no matter the foot type, the majority of weight is borne on the tip of the great toe.[11]

VARIABLE CRITERIA FOR DANCING EN POINTE
Age

No age requirement exists for advancing a dancer to pointe. Dancers need adequate training in technique, however, to attain the skill required to advance. These skills are obtained with years of quality training. Although most female dancers start taking classes at age 4 years,[12] the later years are when the dancers are adequately mature both physically and mentally to acquire and retain the skills and technique required to advance as a dancer. As dancers advance in age, they take an increasing number of ballet classes each week. This repetition is necessary for retention of skill. Usually dancers with years of high-quality training do not attain the skill necessary for pointe until between ages 11 to 13 years. Some dancers may be ready for pointe slightly younger, however, whereas some may be older, and some never may achieve the skill necessary for pointe work.

Growth Plates

Growth occurs at the growth plate, the joint surface, and apophyseal insertions of tendons. These areas of growth are susceptible to injury with overuse, especially during growth spurts.

The growth plates in the feet appear and attain bony maturation at various ages. Some close beyond the age at which dancers first start auditioning and joining professional ballet companies. The base and body of the first metatarsal do not complete ossification until approximately age 18 years to 20 years. Ossification of the phalanges is complete at approximately age 18.[13]

Although only 1 case of premature growth plate closure has been reported in the literature, more may be occurring.[5] The incidence is likely low, however, with little risk to inadequate growth in the long run. Thus, there is no need to wait to start pointe until the growth plates are closed and no need to obtain radiographs to evaluate for growth plate closure to assess for pointe readiness.[14]

Foot Anatomy

Ideally, eventually, a dancer should be able to dance en pointe without pain, injury, or stress. Foot type does not matter for dancing en pointe (**Fig. 3**). Given that most of the weight of dancing en pointe is placed on the first ray, however, the ideal foot type is the peasant or Giselle foot, in which the first 3 toes are of equal length so that the second and third ray may bear some of the weight.[14] Dancers with a Greek

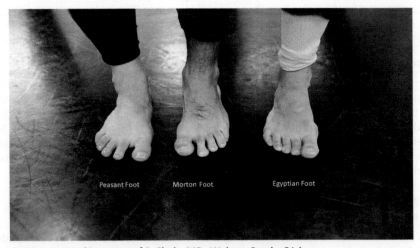

Fig. 3. Foot types. (*Courtesy of* S. Shah, MD, Walnut Creek, CA.)

or Morton foot, in which the second toe is longer than any other, are prone to developing calluses, pain, and hallux rigidis.[14] Dancers with an Egyptian or narrow foot, in which the toe length tapers, may need to add padding to the second toe to help with weight distribution. A dancer with a Simian foot has congenital varus displacement of the first metatarsal and usually has a hypermobile first ray. Dancers with this foot type usually pronate, which often is a precursor to developing a hallux valgus deformity.[15,16]

CRITERIA FOR DANCING EN POINTE
Flexibility

During relevé, the foot should be aligned with the tibia in a straight line for the most ideal position.[17] Much of ballet choreography requires repeated relevés or sustaining a position in relevé, which requires maintaining this alignment throughout. Relevé in ballet slippers requires plantar flexion at the ankle and midfoot and dorsiflexion of the metatarsophalangeal (MTP) joints. Ideally, dancers also have at least 80° to 90° of dorsiflexion in the first MTP joints to achieve proper, full relevé. This perfect rise ideally is developed early on during dance training because it is necessary to train the muscles and the dancer's alignment properly, especially in preparation for pointe.

Dancers must have at least 90° of plantar flexion in the foot and ankle complex to be able to rise en pointe properly.[16] Plantar flexion occurs from the combined motion of the ankle joint, subtalar joint, midtarsal joints, and the MTP joints. In full pointe, the ankle is stable because the subtalar joint is locked between the posterior lip of the tibia and the calcaneus. If a dancer cannot rise fully, she is at risk for injury, especially inversion injuries because the subtalar joint is less stable.[17]

Technique

Turnout
Ideally, ballet dancers are able to turnout or externally rotate their feet to 180°. Dancers often cheat to attain this aesthetic by overpronating the feet, increasing lumbar lordosis, or using excess external tibial torsion.[14] The pointe evaluation is dance based; therefore, it is important to look for improper technique with turnout because this can affect a dancer's ability to develop appropriate strength and proprioception. Flaws should be explained to the dancer during the evaluation so that she can demonstrate the ability to correct the technique and apply them in class moving forward. Also, it is helpful to emphasize to the dancer that controlling turnout is more important than the degree of turnout.

Alignment
Ballet dancers should be able to demonstrate the use of their rhomboid muscles and lower trapezius muscles when holding their arms in the dance positions while demonstrating technique. When raising legs in the various dance positions, the hips ideally should remain parallel to the ground rather than tilting. During turns, the dancer should remain vertical rather than leaning.

Maturity
A dancer must be able to accept corrections, apply them, and remember them. During the evaluation, technique issues should be discussed and recommendations made so that the dancer can demonstrate her ability to apply them and continue using them in class.

Strength

Dancers need strength to be able to sustain positions for a long time, including relevé, especially with legs raised often approximately 90° of hip flexion. Dancers' core muscle strength is imperative for pointe work.

Proprioception

Dancers need to be able sustain holds without quivering and breaking from positions. Before starting pointe, dancers must be able to turn and control their landings with at least 1 single turn on 1 leg.

EVALUATION

The purpose of the 1-on-1 evaluation is multifold: (1) to determine if a dancer is ready for pointe; (2) to serve as an opportunity to discuss and recommend optimal general nutrition and basic health habits, such as sleep hygiene, to optimize the health of the young dancer; and (3) to make recommendations to correct technique that can demonstrate maturity and that can be applied in class moving forward (**Table 1**). Ideally, once the evaluation is complete, a letter or verbal communication with the ballet teacher with documented permission from the dancer and parent is best to review technique flaws that the teacher can help the dancer correct. Often teachers are aware of these, but usually they have several students in class and are unable to point out all of the flaws constantly for each dancer, and the communication can help prioritize the corrections.

The evaluation lasts 1 hour. A parent is required to be present for the entire session for 2 main reasons: (1) the girls are minors and (2) the evaluation serves as an education for the parent about pointe, adequate health habits, and technique issues so that the parent also can help guide the dancer. Dancers should dress as if they are attending class, with their black leotard, pink tights, and hair in a bun. They also should bring their ballet slippers. Some already may have purchased pointe shoes or already may be dancing en pointe, so evaluating the shoes also is beneficial. Since the original publication, the author has added a few additional tests.[17]

History Questions

The history taking is dance and health habit focused. Basic questions include current age, years of dance training, current weekly hours of ballet class and other forms of dance, hours per week of other forms of exercise, and dance goals. Knowing if a dancer wants to continue recreationally versus dance professionally can help when summarizing the evaluation findings at the end, especially for long-term goal setting. The current dance studio is important to know to have an idea of the quality of training as well as any recent studios that a dancer may have switched from. Knowing the main ballet teacher helps facilitate communication regarding the evaluation. Asking what difficulties a dancer notes in class and then what corrections she receives frequently from the teacher is helpful. All dancers receive corrections and a dancer's awareness helps demonstrate maturity. It is important to know about any current injuries because they may affect the evaluation and about any major past injuries that could be affecting the dancer's training. Also, asking about number of hours sleep per night, calcium intake, and vitamin D exposure from sun and supplementation provides an opportunity to make recommendations based on the current age-related health and nutritional guidelines with the goal of preventing bone stress injuries and future osteoporosis.

Table 1		
Shah readiness for pointe evaluation form		
History Questions		**Patient Responses**
Studio name and main ballet teacher		
Age		
Age of first dance class		
Number of years of dance training		
Hours per week of ballet training		
Other forms of dance studied/hours per week		
Other forms of dance studied/hours per week		
Other forms of dance studied/hours per week		
Other forms of dance studied/hours per week		
Other forms of exercise/hours per week		
Dance goals (eg, to become professional ballerina, recreational)		
Difficulties in class (eg, problem with turnout, balance)		
Corrections from teacher		
Past injuries/year/resolved or ongoing		
Current injuries		
Calcium intake		
Vitamin D/sun exposure		
Physical Examination	**Right**	**Left**
Leg length base ASIS to distal tip medial malleolus		
Prone plantar flexion to great toe/to midfoot		
Great toe dorsiflexion degrees		
Prone hip external rotation degrees		
Prone hip internal rotation degrees		
Supine hip external rotation degrees		
Supine hip internal rotation degrees		
Hip external rotation strength		
Hip abduction strength iliotibial band/gluteus medius		
Hip adduction strength leg on top/bottom		
Plantar flexion strength/25 relevés		
Dorsiflexion strength		
Inversion strength		
Eversion strength		
Turnout in first position (compensation) (measure with disk)		
Corrected turnout first position		
Turnout in second position (compensation)		
Turnout in fifth position (compensation)		
Relevé in first (alignment/balance). Hold 5 seconds.		
Relevé second (alignment/balance). Hold 5 seconds.		
Relevé fifth (alignment/balance). Hold 5 seconds.		
Relevé passé each leg (postural control). Hold 5 seconds.		
Lunge (valgus or varus or neutral knee)		

(continued on next page)

Table 1 (continued)		
Physical Examination	Right	Left
Grand plié in first, second, and fifth positions		
Single pirouette each leg (topple test) from fourth position		
Airplane test		
Sauté test		

Assessment and Plan:

Physical Examination

Range of motion and strength

The purpose of the range-of-motion and strength portions of the examination is to determine a dancer's range of motion in the ankle and foot complex and hips as they pertain to dance along with strength. This portion of the examination is helpful in determining why a dancer may not be ready for pointe and explaining what a dancer needs to work on to help develop the needed skills. Often, there are differences between left and right and these should be discussed and summarized at the end of the evaluation.

Leg length differences can affect a dancer's ability to properly achieve alignment, so this can be pointed out as well for a dancer to work on and helps her understand why she may be struggling more on 1 side than the other. Even if a dancer is ready for pointe, usually there are some deficits that can be discussed with the dancer to help her optimize training. Leg length is measured from the anterior superior iliac spine (ASIS) to the medial malleolus and should be done consistently on each side from tip to tip.

Various angle measurements are taken with a goniometer. Prone plantar flexion is measured to ensure that the dancer has the required 90° of plantar flexion to go en pointe. Great toe dorsiflexion is measured next. If it is less than 80° and a dancer does not rise to full demi-pointe relevé during the examination, this can be reviewed with her and perhaps can be improved with safe stretching techniques or further evaluation recommended to determine if there is an anatomic issue. Hip external and internal rotations are evaluated supine and prone to determine if there are left and right differences that may be affecting a dancer's turnout more on 1 side then the other.

Hip strength is checked on the examination table. Hip abduction strength testing is done by testing the gluteus medius and tensor fascia lata separately, because the author has found that the gluteus medius often is weak and dancers benefit from focused strengthening. Hip adduction is checked with the leg on top and on the bottom side lying. Ankle strength, including dorsiflexion, plantar flexion, inversion, and eversion, is checked while the dancer is seated with the leg hanging down. Plantar flexion is assessed further by asking the dancer to perform 25 relevés on each leg with the arms crossed on the chest. Dancers are asked to stop when they feel fatigued or are visibly fatigued. Strength is assigned in increments of 5 successful relevés with a 5/5 given if a dancer can perform all 25, 4/5 for 20, and so on, with 1/5 if she can perform only 5.

Successful passage of the airplane test is imperative (**Fig. 4**).[18] This test is performed by standing on 1 leg with the arms at 180° to the side and trunk outstretched forward and the opposite leg extended posteriorly to create a 180° line while balancing on the standing leg to create a T-shaped position. Then, the dancer performs 5

Airplane Test Starting Position   **Airplane Test Ending Position**

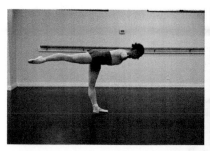
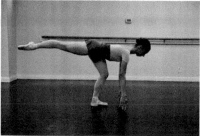

Fig. 4. Airplane test. (*Courtesy of* S. Shah, MD, Walnut Creek, CA.)

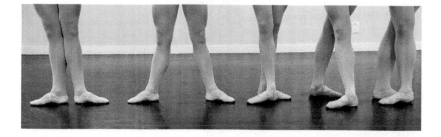

First Position   Second Position   Third Position   Fourth Position Fifth Position

Fig. 5. Five basic positions of ballet. (*Courtesy of* S. Shah, MD, Walnut Creek, CA.)

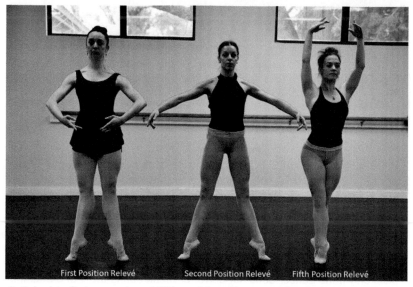

First Position Relevé   Second Position Relevé   Fifth Position Relevé

Fig. 6. Relevé in first, second, and fifth position. (*Courtesy of* S. Shah, MD, Walnut Creek, CA.)

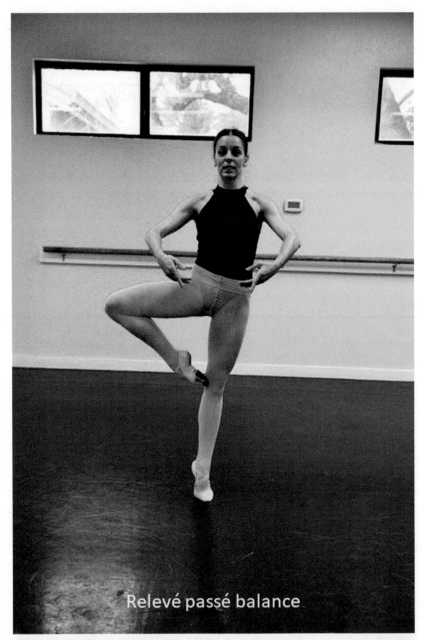

Relevé passé balance

Fig. 7. Relevé passé balance. (*Courtesy of* S. Shah, MD, Walnut Creek, CA.)

controlled pliés (bend at the knee keeping the foot flat on the ground) while horizontally adducting the arms to touch the finger tips to the ground. A pass is defined as greater than or equal to 4 of 5 pliés, maintaining neutral alignment.[18] The author allows a complete pass only if the dancer does not quiver or break during the 4 of 5 attempts for each leg. If the dancer does quiver or sway and is able to complete the series, however, this is noted and taken into account during the final assessment.

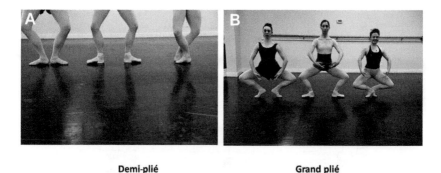

Demi-plié   **Grand plié**

Fig. 8. Demi-plié and grand plié. (*Courtesy of* S. Shah, MD, Walnut Creek, CA.)

Dance-based and functional assessment

Turnout is measured in first position, ideally standing on disks that a dancer stands on to measure turnout so that a dancer can understand what her natural turnout is. There are 5 basic positions in dance (**Fig. 5**) and turnout is assessed in first, second, and fifth positions because they are used most commonly in ballet class. With any of the fifth position assessments, both right in front of left and left in front of right should be evaluated. During the turnout assessment any inappropriate compensations, or cheating, as discussed previously, should be reviewed. This gives the dancer an opportunity to correct and demonstrate her ability to apply corrections, which can continue to be monitored during the rest of the assessment.

Relevé is assessed in first, second, and fifth positions (**Fig. 6**). The dancer should be able to hold each position for 5 seconds, holding the arms in first position (arms slightly rounded and forward flexed to approximately 80°) without quivering or breaking to pass.

Relevé passé balance is assessed on each side. A dancer must be able to stand on 1 leg, with the gesture leg flexed at the knee with the toe touching the standing knee and hip in external rotation and flexion (**Fig. 7**). The dancer can start by holding on to a ballet barre, wall, or table to get the balance and then let go of the support. The dancer should be able to balance in this position on relevé for 5 seconds with arms in first position without quivering or breaking to pass.

Grand plié is evaluated in first, second, and fifth positions (**Fig. 8**). Grand plié is performed by first doing demi-plié (see **Fig. 8**A) and then bending further to a squat in each position so that the heels are raised as in a relevé position squat (see **Fig. 8**B).

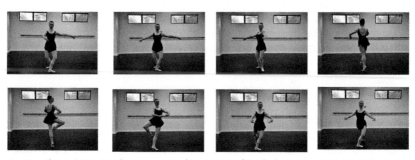

Fig. 9. Fourth position single pirouette. (*Courtesy of* S. Shah, MD, Walnut Creek, CA.)

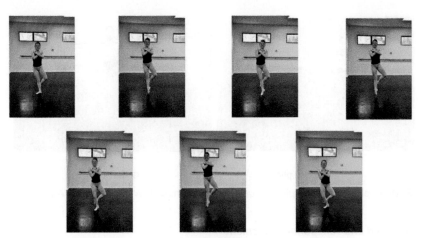

Fig. 10. State 3 Sauté jumps using still photography. (*Courtesy of* S. Shah, MD, Walnut Creek, CA.)

Dancers should be able to perform this using the arm motions in dance without leaning forward or swaying.

Standing lunges are performed to evaluate for neutral, valgus, or varus knee alignment when landing the lunge. Issues should be reviewed with the patient. Dancers with valgus landings may be at risk for anterior knee pain and also difficulties with maintaining balance.

The topple test is single-leg pirouette turn performed from fourth position.[18] The dancer turns with the leg in a passé position. The dancer must be able to perform a controlled turn and land without swaying or breaking and landing back in fourth position (**Fig. 9**).

The sauté, or jump, test is performed on each leg with the arms across the chest.[18] The other leg is elevated with the foot in a coupe position: ankle plantar flexed or pointed at the ankle (**Fig. 10**). A dancer should be able to perform 8 of 16 jumps with proper alignment and control (staying in 1 place; no sway, lean, or break; and able to jump high enough to plantar flex the standing foot in midair).

Formulating the Assessment

At the end of the evaluation, the health practitioner should summarize the findings and make recommendations regarding health habit improvements and technique, strength, and alignment corrections. Ideally, it is best to provide a series of strengthening exercise handouts based on findings and, if possible, refer to a physical therapist and/or Pilates instructor who specializes in dance to work with the dancer. Based on the examination, a dancer either may be ready to advance for pointe immediately or may need to work on some areas and be re-evaluated at a time the health practitioner feels is appropriate.

SUMMARY

Advancing to pointe requires sufficient maturity, strength, and flexibility and adequate ballet training to develop necessary skills, including proper technique, alignment, and balance. Health practitioners can help studios determine if dancers are ready to advance to pointe by providing an objective assessment. In addition to determining if a dancer is ready to advance to pointe, the evaluation provides an opportunity for the health practitioner to make suggestions to help optimize the dancer's health and improve the dancer's technique. The physical examination portion is largely dance based, making it critical for health practitioners to familiarize themselves with ballet technique to be able to make an appropriate determination.

One study showed that the airplane test, sauté test, and topple test correlated with advancing to pointe based on the teachers' assessment in the study serving as the gold standard. This may not necessarily be applicable to all dancers, however, given the wide variability among studios, and these tests alone do not provide information as to why a dancer may be struggling.[18]

Many dance medicine practitioners use a variety of screening tools, based on previous articles published or creating their own using a conglomeration of tests. The recommended evaluation in this article not only allows determining if a dancer is ready for pointe but also allows the health practitioner to find the problem areas and make suggestions for corrections for a dancer to work on to either become ready eventually or improve a dancer's technique if she is ready. The future goal is to validate this screen and then determine if there is a reduction in injuries and discomfort in those dancers who go en pointe who are passed by using this screen versus those who go en pointe despite a recommendation against starting en pointe or delaying the start based on this screen.

DISCLOSURE

The author has no financial or commercial conflicts of interest.

REFERENCES

1. Hardaker WT, Vander Woude LM. Dance medicine: an orthopaedist's view. N C Med J 1993;43:67–72.
2. Barringer J, Schlesinger S. The pointe book. Pennington (NJ): Princeton Book Company; 1991. p. 1–3.
3. Bickle C, Deighan M, Theis N. The effect of pointe shoe deterioration on foot and ankle kinematics and kinetics in professional ballet dancers. Hum Mov Sci 2018; 60:72–7.
4. Aquino J, Amasay T, Shapiro S, et al. Lower Extremity biomechanics and muscle activity differ between "new" and "dead" pointe shoes in professiona ballet dancers. Sports Biomech 2019;1–12.
5. Shah S. Premature Growth Plate Closure in a Ballet Dancer *en Pointe*. Clin J Sport Med 2017;27(5):e69–71.
6. Davenport K, Simmel L, Kadel N. Hallux Valgus in Dancers: A Closer Look at Dance Technique and Its Impact on Dancers' Feet. J Dance Med Sci 2010; 18(2):86–92.
7. Steinberg N, Siev-Ner I, Peleg S, et al. Injuries in Female Dancers Aged 8 – 16. J Athl Train 2013;48(1):118–23.
8. Lee L, Reid D, Cadwell J. Injury Incidence, Dance Exposure and the Use of the Movement Competency Screen (MCS) to Identify Variables Associated with Injury in Full-time Pre-Professional Dancers. Int J Sports Phys Ther 2017;12(3):352–70.
9. Pearson S, Whitaker A. Footwear in Classical Ballet: A Study of Pressure Distribution and Related Foot Injury in the Adolescent Dancer. J Dance Med Sci 2012; 16(2):51–6.
10. Meck C, Hess R, Helldobler R, et al. Pre-Pointe Evaluation Components Used by Dance Schools. J Dance Med Sci 2004;8(2):37–42.

11. Teitz CC, Harrington RM, Wiley H. Pressures on the Foot in Pointe Shoes. Foot Ankle 1985;5(5):216–21.
12. Young C, Shah S, Gottschlich L. Dance. In: Madden C, Putukian M, Young C, et al, editors. Netter sports medicine. 2nd edition. Philadelphia: Elsevier; 2017. p. 693–9.
13. Gray H. Anatomy of the human body. Philadelphia: Lea & Febiger; 2000.
14. Ogilve-Harris D, Carr M, Fleming P. The Foot in Ballet Dancers: the Importance of Second Toe Length. Foot Ankle Int 1995;16:144–7.
15. Hamilton WG. Ballet. In: Reider B, editor. Sports medicine, the school-age athete. Philadelphia: W.B. Saunders Company; 1996.
16. Shah S. Caring for the Dancer: Special Considerations for the Performer and Troupe. Curr Sports Med Rep 2008;7(3):128–32.
17. Shah S. Determining a Young Dancer's Readiness for Pointe. Curr Sports Med Rep 2009;8(6):295–9.
18. Richardson M, Liederbach M, Sandow E. Functional criteria for assessing pointe-readiness. J Dance Med Sci 2010;14(3):82–8.

Choreography-Specific Cross-Training and Conditioning Programs

Emma Faulkner, PT, DPT, OCS

KEYWORDS

- Cross-training • Conditioning • Dance injury • Specificity of training

KEY POINTS

- Traditional ballet class does not challenge the aerobic capacity of a dancer enough to create training adaptations.
- Additional cardiovascular conditioning and cross-training programs are beneficial for dancers.
- Exercise and sport science principles can and should be applied to dancers for performance enhancement and injury prevention.
- Specificity of training to the level of specific choreography demands can improve dancer's performance, artistry, and safety.

INTRODUCTION

Dance is generally considered to be an amalgam of art and athletics, with a greater emphasis historically on the artistic component. Dance performance requires significant athletic fitness and physiologic capacity, but also requires the finesse, storytelling, and creativity of an art form. When looking at sports literature, dance is generally not included in the list of sports, although there is little argument that dancers are required to have similar physical attributes as athletes in other sports. Athletes in any sport must possess some degree of muscular strength and endurance, anaerobic and aerobic metabolic efficiency, speed, agility, coordination, motor control, balance, and psychological preparedness in order to perform adequately in his or her respective sport. Each sport will require different ratios of each of these characteristics and, as a result, training will need to be designed to meet the particular needs of the specific sport. Similarly, each genre of dance requires specific training to meet its unique goals.

The term "athlete" is a generic term that provides little detail into the physical capacity or quality of sport performance. For example, a rugby player and a marathoner are both

Atlanta Ballet, Atlanta Dance Medicine, TriHealth Physical Therapy, LLC, Department of Theater and Dance, Emory University, 215 Church Street Suite 101, Decatur, GA 30030, USA
E-mail address: emma@trihealthphysicaltherapy.com

Phys Med Rehabil Clin N Am 32 (2021) 103–115
https://doi.org/10.1016/j.pmr.2020.09.003

defined as athletes but will look different and demonstrate different proportions of muscular strength, cardiorespiratory endurance, and sport-specific motor control. The term "dancer" is equally as generic as "athlete." A "dancer" can be trained in ballet, modern, jazz, hip hop, tap, Irish dance, Highland dance, or any of the traditional African, Chinese, Indian, or other dance forms that have specific geographic origins. Each of these dancers will look and perform with a different movement vocabulary that places emphasis on different physiologic attributes. For example, a classical ballet dancer will often perform in pointe shoes with leaps, turns, and high leg holds, whereas, in the traditional Indian style of Bharatnatyam, the dancer flexes the bare foot and maintains a flexed knee position throughout most of the dance performance. Each of these performers is considered a "dancer" but will undergo different training regimens and will demonstrate different injury patterns. Although it is important to provide specificity regarding the type of athlete being trained, it is also important to understand the genre of dance being performed with its specific movement demands in order to develop appropriate conditioning and cross-training for optimal dance performance and injury prevention.

DANCERS AS PERFORMING ATHLETES

Physiologically, dance performance is a highly skilled, moderate- to high-intensity, intermittently performed activity.[1] In order to carry out this activity at the highest level, dancers must maintain high levels of physical fitness and physiologic conditioning, in addition to exceptional levels of technical skill in their specific dance genre. Training programs for dance are currently based on tradition and routine with the emphasis on imagery and the final aesthetic of the movement performance rather than the anatomic or muscular requirement needed to achieve final performance.

From early training, which can begin as young as 3 or 4 years old, skill acquisition and perfection of movement are often predominant goals of the dance training program, regardless of genre.[2] Throughout the lifetime of a dancer's training, there is less focus on the development of overall physical capacity or cardiovascular endurance for the purpose of increased skill acquisition or improved performance. In sport, training programs are scientifically based to create the desired performance response, which uses sport-appropriate energy systems and often leads to an underlying level of general physical preparedness among the 3 metabolic energy systems.[3] A significant difference in the training methodologies between dance and sport is that preparation for performance will occur regardless of a dancer's overall physical fitness level. Because of the young age of training initiation, dancers often become specialized earlier than their sport counterparts.[4] Early sport specialization has been demonstrated to correlate with increased injury and early sport drop out.[5] This early specialization, in conjunction with minimal overall fitness training, could be correlated to the increased incidence of overuse injuries in the dance population, especially among adolescents and trainees.[6]

In professional ballet, a dancer generally begins the day with ballet class for 60 to 90 minutes. This class is often a traditional ballet class with warmup by holding on to the barre and then progressing to the center of the room with slow controlled movements, followed by jumping, and then possibly a short performance combination of different movement elements. Research into the energy systems used in a ballet class has shown that the class is overall minimally aerobic, unlike dance performance, and the physiologic challenge begins once the dancer moves from the barre to the center.[7,8] Following class, the professional dancer generally will have rehearsal for the upcoming performances. Rehearsals on a full day can last up to 6 hours and are highly variable in intensity.

The traditional ballet class is the primary form of training for dance performance, but there are inconsistencies between energy requirements during class and during performance. Higher intensities of activity are required during performance but are not adequately trained during the lower-intensity classes used as preparation. Research conducted by Wyon and Redding[2] into the energy requirements for ballet class, rehearsals, and performance has found significant differences among the 3 settings. Within class itself, there have been differences found between the warmup/barre portion and the center portion.[3,8,9] During the center phase of class, which more closely resembles performance, the work-to-rest ratio heavily favored rest.[10] The intensity measures reported in this research demonstrated that the center portion was moderate to high intensity.[2,7–10] Comparing this class data to the performance data, the differences become even more apparent. Research concludes that dance performance is high-intensity intermittent activity that relies on both the aerobic and the anaerobic energy pathways.

Although Wyon and Redding compared energy requirements during class versus performance, research conducted by Rodrigues-Krause and colleagues[11] in Brazil studied the physiologic requirements of isolated sets of ballet exercises performed during class. This study found that Vo_2 values are lower during the barre exercises at the beginning of class and higher during center exercises, which have been described as moderate to high intensity.[3,10] This research correlates Vo_2 numerical values to the intensities during each section of class described by Wyon and Redding.[2]

Underscoring the findings of both Wyon and Rodriguez, it has been found that dancers have similar maximal oxygen uptake values (Vo_{2max}) as healthy sedentary adults, indicating a lack of adequate aerobic cardiovascular training during a dancer's typical genre-specific dance training regimen (ie, ballet class).[2,12] Furthermore, few professional ballet companies exclusively perform classical ballet works. Most ballet companies are mixed repertoire companies, which means that classically trained ballet dancers may be expected to dance classical, contemporary modern, or highly stylized choreography. Regardless of the genre, style, or intensity of the pieces being rehearsed, the ballet class, which is the primary training regimen for the dancer, still follows the classical and traditional format.[1,13] Therefore, it has been almost universally recommended that dancers supplement their dance technique training with additional aerobic exercise. Because of the intermittent nature of dance, steady state cardiovascular endurance exercise is not considered to be the most effective way for a dancer to improve aerobic capacity. Instead, interval training is an effective way for dancers to more closely resemble the work-to-rest ratios common in class and performance. The intervals can be manipulated depending on training goals, choreographic requirements, and prior physical fitness level.

DANCE INJURY

In dance, as with all sports or physical activities, injuries are prevalent and often specific to the dance genre. With the shift to recognizing dancers as athletes, there has been more research completed regarding injury tracking, incidence, prevention, and treatment. Musculoskeletal injury is an inherent risk with any physical activity, and generally, the risk and incidence of injury increase with increased difficulty of the activity and with increased time participating in the activity. Dance injury research, as a whole, has suggested that the general physical fitness level in most dancers is not adequate, and as a result, many dancers suffer significant injuries and performance deficits.[1,10,12,14] The advancements in dance research has brought up concerns that the focus on science and physicality could negatively impact the aesthetic and artistic elements of dance as an art form.[1,13] Unlike traditional sports, many genres of dance are steeped in tradition, artistry, communication, and storytelling.[15] Tradition not only influences performance of these dance forms but also provides the basis for a dancer's training. Only recently, dancers have started to recognize the significance of emphasizing athletic and physiologic components of dance to enhance artistry rather than detract from it.[12]

Dance injury has been the topic of research, but the operational definition of a "dance injury" has not been unified throughout this research.[16] It is important that researchers agree on how to define the term "injury" because systematic reviews demonstrate injury rates anywhere from 40% to 94% in professional dancers and show that upwards of 95% of professional dancers report musculoskeletal pain in some capacity.[4,17,18] Although recent research has attempted to more accurately define dance injury using time loss or a functional/participatory loss in the injury definition,[9,10] there still is significant discrepancy in the literature, which makes reporting true injury rates challenging. Despite the variable definitions, it is clear that injuries are prevalent in recreational[19,20] through professional[21-26] settings of all dance genres.[19,21,22,27-31] **Table 1** demonstrates the range of injury incidence values (per 1000 exposure hours) and varying injury definitions in selected studies of youth through professional ballet dancers. Another commonality in dance injury research is that overuse injuries are more prevalent than traumatic injuries,[25,30,32] although some gender[20,30] and genre[27] differences have been reported. Consistently, this dance injury research has demonstrated that higher injury rates typically correlate with increased dance exposures.[33,34]

Injury risk factors and prevention programs are heavily explored in dance medicine and science literature. Researchers, dancers, and directors agree that some of the most significant risk factors for dance injury can be broken down into 3 categories: physiologic, technical, and environmental.[22] Physiologic risk factors include age, anatomic variations, nutritional status, levels of fatigue, and muscle

Table 1
Injury definition and incidence rate in ballet dancers

Study	Population Studied	Injury Definition	Injury Incidence Rate
Ramkumar et al,[26] 2016	Single professional ballet company, 10-y retrospective study	Medical and time loss	0.91/1000 h
Allen et al,[24] 2013	Single company professional dancers, 3-y prospective study	Time-loss	1.71–4.4/1000 h over 3-y study period
Nilsson et al,[25] 2001	Swedish professional ballet company over 5 y	Medical (orthopedic)	0.6/1000 h
Gamboa et al,[31] 2008	Preprofessional ballet dancers in an elite training program (age 9–20)	Treatment (physical therapy)	1.09/1000 h
Leanderson et al,[20] 2011	Youth ballet students aged 10–21	Medical (orthopedic)	0.3–1.1/1000 h
Ekegren et al,[34] 2014	Preprofessional ballet dancers aged 16–19	Medical and time loss	1.38/1000 h

Data from Refs [20,24-26,31,34].

imbalance. The relationship between fatigue levels and injury risk is gaining recognition as a significant risk factor because of the growing physical demands of today's choreography.[1,3,35] Some of these risk factors can be decreased with appropriate intervention to manage the risk and promote increased physical preparedness for dance. Environmental risk factors, such as stage or flooring materials, lighting, and shoe wear, may be adjusted, to an extent, to decrease risk of injury.[21] Technical risk factors are one of the most easily mitigated. Proper training, teaching dancers to move safely within the limits of their anatomy, and appropriate cross-training or conditioning programs to improve overall strength and physical fitness can all assist in improving technique to decrease injury. Most injury-prevention programs are aimed at mitigating one or more of these risk factors and are completed at a company-wide level. Additional research has shown an increased benefit of personalized injury-prevention programs that take into consideration the individual dancer's past injury history and scores on standardized functional measures.[24]

EXERCISE PHYSIOLOGY PRINCIPLES APPLIED TO DANCE

Three commonly studied exercise science principles that apply to basic physical training and enhancing training adaptations include *specificity of training*, *overload*, and *periodization*. Each of these training principles needs to be considered when developing any exercise program, regardless of mode of exercise or training goals.

Specificity of Training

Specificity of training refers to "the body's physiologic and metabolic responses and adaptations to exercise are specific to the type of exercise and muscle groups involved."[36] Specificity of training, in essence, is a response elicited by training in the specific mode of exercise that is to be performed. Strength and conditioning coach Paul Gamble[37] further breaks down the principle of specificity into metabolic specificity, biomechanical specificity, and psychological specificity. Metabolic specificity adaptations occur when the same metabolic pathways that are necessary for performance are specifically used during training. This subcategory of specificity is the section that has been most closely addressed in the dance medicine literature. Significant research has studied energy utilization during different sections of class, rehearsal, and performance.[2,8–11,38] This work could assist in developing a framework for a training program for metabolic specificity in the ballet and contemporary dance genres.[2,10] By understanding the work-to-rest ratios in different components of class, as well as different selected exercises within ballet as discussed previously in research by Rodrigues-Krause and colleagues,[11] it can be determined that interval training is preferred when developing supplemental training for ballet and contemporary dancers. Because of the differences in work-to-rest ratios between classes, rehearsals, and performance, it is evident that ballet class alone is not the single or the most appropriate training mode for dance performance. Conditioning and cross-training programs performed in intervals can be manipulated to mimic the work-to-rest ratio that the dancer needs during a performance.

The second subcategory of the specificity principle discussed by Gamble[37] is biomechanical specificity. Training effects and adaptations are due to the specific type, speed, pattern, and strength of muscle contraction. This type of specificity can assist a dancer in skill acquisition as well as development of muscular strength, endurance, and power. Of particular note in a dancer population are the extreme ranges of motion (ROM) that are required to perform many dance movements. The heavily studied genres of ballet and contemporary demonstrate excess ROM requirements at the foot, ankle,[31,38] and hip.[39,40]

Excess ROM or extreme flexibility of the joints and soft tissues can be described as "hypermobility" and can be hereditary, developed through dance training, or a combination of both factors. Many dancers demonstrate a combination of both, which results in the flexibility needed to excel in technical dance movements. Hypermobility, or greater than average flexibility, is a trait often desired by artistic directors, dance instructors, choreographers, and dancers themselves when determining if a dancer has the potential to become a professional.[39] Training for dance-specific strength and muscle endurance requires specific exercises for strength and motor control that work within the required end ROM for dance. There are few traditional sports that require a specific exercise for training the hip flexor group at a flexion range of greater than 100° for an isometric hold, but this movement is practiced daily in ballet. Often, general strength training exercises (ie, squat, dead lift, calf raise) may not challenge the full ROM required to perform as a professional dancer. **Fig. 1** demonstrates the ROM differences between a traditional calf raise and the ballet demi pointe position, and **Fig. 2** demonstrates the ROM differences between a bodyweight squat and a ballet grande plié. Dancers must include specific variations of traditional exercises to work into their end ROM and develop dance-specific biomechanical training adaptations.

The final subcategory of specificity of training that Gamble[37] discusses is the principle of psychological specificity. This subsection would be even more significant in a dance training program because of the artistic nature of the activity. The purpose behind movement and the intention is what creates the communication and storytelling necessary for dance performance. Two key ideas within psychological specificity are mental effort and intent. In a sport like baseball, often the intent behind a "run" is to get the athlete to a goal or end point faster than opponents or the ball. In dance, a "run" can be used functionally to get a dancer from 1 point on the stage to another, but

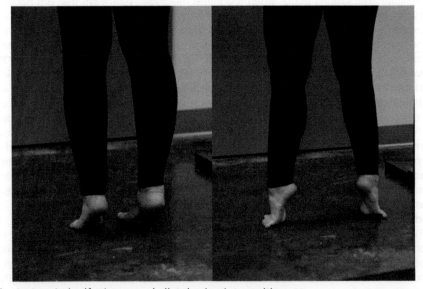

Fig. 1. A typical calf raise versus ballet demi pointe position.

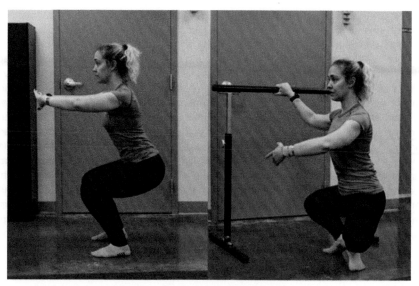

Fig. 2. A body weight squat versus first position grande plié.

usually there is an intent behind the "run" that is important to the storyline. The "run" can be toward a lover, away from something fear inducing, or jovial and spritely to communicate the idea of being youthful and carefree. Each of those intentions produces a different running mechanic that needs to be specifically addressed. Because dancers are precision athletes who must demonstrate emotion through their physicality, training them for safe and high-level execution of extraordinary skills is critical, as is training the dancer for a specific performance, role, or character so they can create the art.

Overload Principle

The *overload principle* explains that in order for training adaptations to occur and improvements to be made in any physical fitness component, the physiologic systems used during an athlete's preferred activity must be trained at a level greater than the athlete is accustomed. Overload can occur by manipulating variables of training, including speed, load, intensity, or duration of activity.[36,41] The principle of overload is one that most dancers are familiar with. Often dancers are pushing past limits, pushing their bodies to extremes, and performing hundreds of repetitions of movements in an attempt to achieve relative perfection. In some instances, this overload leads to overuse and injuries, especially in the lower extremities because of high-impact stress from jumps. In a single 90-minute ballet class, dancers can perform upwards of 200 jumps with more than half of these landing on a single lower extremity.[42] Although dancers often overload their bodies mechanically, they do not often overload their cardiovascular systems.[1–3,7,8,10–12] Using overload to improve cardiovascular fitness and improve the efficiency of metabolic energy pathways would be an appropriate application of this principle for dancers.

Periodization Principle

Periodization is an important principle in sport but is less frequently studied or used within dance. Periodization systematically varies the intensity and/or volume of training in order to promote training adaptations to the neuromuscular system and to minimize the detrimental effect of overtraining.[36] In sports with distinct training seasons, off-seasons, and competition seasons, each with different intensities and goals, periodization is inherently built in. Dance does not have a specific "off-season" so periodization must be used strategically year round to achieve the desired training adaptations and prevent overtraining.[43] For adolescent and student dancers, there really is no true off- season. These dancers work through the academic year at their dance schools and then often travel for summer intensives, which, as their name implies, are often more intense than the normal dance schedule. Once summer is over, these students are back to their home studios and typical dance/school routines without any significant break. In professional dance companies, contracts are generally 25 to 40 weeks long. Professional dancers often have a lighter summer off-season, although many professional dancers teach or continue to perform as guest artists during this time. This schedule does not allow for ramp-up or ramp-down of training. The dance world needs to consider integrating the principle of periodization into a training schedule that addresses the needs of a dancer during both rehearsal and performance periods.

CHOREOGRAPHY-SPECIFIC PROGRAMMING

Many researchers have recommended the utilization of science and sport training principles for dancers.[12,13,21,44] Some professional dance companies and training programs have begun to develop specific conditioning programs and provide onsite training facilities for their dancers.[45,46] These programs and facilities are vital for assisting dancers in the development of general physical preparedness, rehabilitating injuries, and participating in dance-specific training programs. Most of the public-access dance training programs are basic conditioning programs, ballet-specific programs, or programs developed by dance-specific personal trainers or dance physiotherapists. Although excellent, many programs lack the detailed specificity that today's professional company dancer needs. Most large ballet companies and contemporary ballet companies are required to perform in multiple styles and genres of dance, sometimes within the same evening's performance. Because of the choreographic variability and steadily increasing choreographic challenges, there needs to be a push toward even more specificity of training to enhance performance for the required choreography. This level of specificity would be akin to training pitchers, catchers, and outfielders for their specific positions rather than just giving each member of a baseball or softball team a generic "baseball or softball" conditioning program. Specificity of training seems like common sense when looked at through the sport lens but has yet to become commonplace in the dance world.

The development and implementation of a choreography-specific training program should be a collaborative effort between the choreographer/stager and the medical team or trainer. This collaboration will allow both parties to understand the demands being placed on the dancer during the performance as well as the physical requirements needed to create the desired performance aesthetic. When developing a choreography-specific program, factors to consider are the length of the choreography, intensity of the choreography, and metabolic energy demands. The work-to-rest ratio of dancers often correlates to the time on stage versus off stage, but in some instances, dancers may be on stage with low-energy demand but for an extended period. For example, the energy demands for the same time on stage between the corps de ballet (balancing in the background) and a principal dancer (completing jumps in front) may be drastically different performing the same classical ballet. Many classical ballets are cast by rank, and it is important to consider specificity for each dancer's choreography and not the ballet as a whole. In this example, stage time for each dancer is important, but more important are the choreography demands for each role. Increased training in all 3 subcategories of specificity for each dancer and each specific role should theoretically prepare the dancer for the athleticism as well as the artistry to allow performance at the highest level.

The format of a conditioning program should be similar to the requirements of performance with respect to intensity, metabolic pathway utilization, work-to-rest ratios, and biomechanical movement requirements. A case example would be the training program developed at a professional ballet company to train dancers for a specific contemporary piece, Ohad Naharin's *Minus 16*, which uses an entirely different movement vocabulary from classical ballet, called Gaga. This movement vocabulary was developed by Naharin and was designed to push the limits of dancers past familiar limits. When asked in an interview to describe his movement, Naharin stated that he did not like to define it as "classical," "high art," "street," "modern," or "hip hop," but he wanted to "abolish recognition… take form and take content and put it in a blender."[47]

In the *Minus 16* example, the training program was developed by a physical therapist (PT), with prior professional dance experience who worked for the ballet company, and the ballet mistress who was responsible for rehearsing and staging the work. This company saw a need for this training program following prior seasons' performances of *Minus 16*, which resulted in specific injuries, primarily cervical spine, shoulder, and lumbar spine, directly related to the piece. *Minus 16* as Naharin hoped "abolishes recognition." It is not a classical ballet; it is not a contemporary ballet. There are elements of comedy, contemporary dance, and improvisation with extensive onstage costume changes, dancing with props, and audience participation, which makes it unlike other works performed by classical ballet companies today.

During the development of the program, the PT and the ballet mistress learned the choreography in order to intimately understand what was required for its performance. It was during this time that the PT reviewed treatment notes from the prior seasons' performances and interviewed dancers regarding which parts of the dance they thought resulted in which injuries. The section of the dance that was identified as most taxing to the dancers and posing the highest injury risk is the performance of repetitive movements in canon while sitting in chairs that form a semicircle around the stage. These phrases are sharp, technical, explosive, dynamic, and eventually result in the last dancer repeatedly thrusting their body out of the chair and collapsing onto the ground.[48] Because the work required short, high-intensity phrases followed by pauses and stillness in the chairs, a high-intensity interval training program (HIIT) using a Tabata-style protocol was used. This style of HIIT training developed by Japanese researcher Dr Izumi Tabata was found to improve both the anaerobic and the aerobic metabolic energy systems.[49] Timing from the phrases in the work was used to determine the intervals that would most replicate the work-to-rest ratios the dancers experience while performing. The movements designed for the intervals were developed by the PT and the ballet mistress. The psychological specificity and intention of the movement were described by the ballet mistress using the vocabulary of this specific dance style and contemporary dance terms. The phrases were broken down into specific biomechanical movements to determine muscle patterning, initiation points, and possible risks for injury. Together with the understanding of the metabolic, biomechanical, and psychological specifics that *Minus 16* requires, the PT and the ballet mistress created a unique interval training program with additional strengthening exercises to address areas of concern within the movement.

Dancers voluntarily participated in the programming before the performance of the piece. Most dancers took part in the programming 2 to 3 times per week when out of their performance season and once or twice weekly during their performance season. During the final weeks leading up to the performance of *Minus 16*, the dancers stopped the additional exercise programming to focus on rehearsals and prepare for performances without overloading their bodies. When describing this aspect of timing the exercise program to the dancers, the PT described the sport concept of a nonlinear periodization program,[24] such as in weightlifting as a "deload" or in distance running as a "taper."[43,50]

Anecdotally, the company had less injury directly related to the performance of *Minus 16* than they had in prior seasons' performances. In addition, when interviewed, dancers described the performance differently following participation in the training program. They, as a whole, felt more prepared and stronger in the movement style, which they thought was related to their participation in the specific training program for this piece of choreography.[51]

Although this is only 1 example of implementing a program for a specific piece of choreography, it does provide encouraging results. Because the sample size was small and only select members of 1 professional company participated, no generalizations can be made or direct conclusions that this method of training is the optimal way to train. What this case example does show is that this method of training has potential benefits that could be expanded upon if additional development and implementation of similar programs continue to take place in professional companies. It is hoped not only that eventually a dance company would not only have a reparatory of dance choreography to perform in a given season but also that each piece would be accompanied by a specific training program to optimize dancer wellness and performance while performing a specific choreography.

DISCUSSION

As is seen in professional sports, often there is a trickle-down effect from professional programs into the adolescent or recreational programs. One could anticipate the same trickle-down effect occurring from the professional ballet companies down to the preprofessional schools and training programs. This earlier start of highly specified conditioning and cross-training has the potential to alter injury patterns throughout the spectrum of dance abilities. It could also be extrapolated to additional genres of dance. It could be hypothesized that because younger dancers often participate in multiple genres of dance, the specificity of training for each type of performance would be highly beneficial for performance quality and injury prevention.

Because of increased choreographic demands, early specialization, multi-genre dancers, and high incidence of career-ending injuries, there is a need for enhanced training methodologies to address the unique needs of today's professional dancer. It is imperative for company directors, instructors, choreographers, and dance medicine practitioners to consider implementing the most specific conditioning and training programs to prepare their dancers to meet or exceed expectations without resultant injury. Quantifying effectiveness of choreography-specific training programs is an area for further research. Now that most of the world can agree that dancers are athletes and dance is not solely an art form, the vast scientific knowledge base that applies to fitness, sport, and athletics should be explored more thoroughly in dance. The implementation of scientific principles can and should be used to enhance dancers' health, performance, athleticism, and artistry.

DISCLOSURE

The author has nothing to disclose.

REFERENCES

1. Koutedakis Y, Jamurtas A. The dancer as a performing athlete: physiological considerations. Sports Med 2004;34(10):651–61.
2. Wyon MA, Redding E. Physiological monitoring of cardiorespiratory adaptations during rehearsal and performance of contemporary dance. J Strength Cond Res 2005;19(3):611–4.
3. Beck S, Redding E, Wyon MA. Methodological considerations for documenting the energy demand of dance activity: a review. Front Psychol 2015;6:568.
4. Hincapié CA, Morton EJ, Cassidy JD. Musculoskeletal injuries and pain in dancers: a systematic review. Arch Phys Med Rehabil 2008;89(9):1819–29.
5. Jayanthi NA, LaBella CR, Fischer D, et al. Sports-specialized intensive training and the risk of injury in young athletes: a clinical case-control study. Am J Sports Med 2015;43(4):794–801.
6. Sugimoto D, Jackson SS, Howell DR, et al. Association between training volume and lower extremity overuse injuries in young female athletes: implications for early sports specialization. Phys Sportsmed 2019;47(2):199–204.
7. Kozai AC, Twitchett E, Morgan S, et al. Workload intensity and rest periods in professional ballet: connotations for injury. Int J Sports Med 2020;41(6):373–9.
8. Rodrigues-Krause J, Krause M, Reischak-Oliveira Á. Cardiorespiratory considerations in dance: from classes to performances. J Dance Med Sci 2015;19(3): 91–102.
9. Rodrigues-Krause J, Krause M, Cunha Gdos S, et al. Ballet dancers cardiorespiratory, oxidative and muscle damage responses to classes and rehearsals. Eur J Sport Sci 2014;14(3):199–208.
10. Twitchett EA, Koutedakis Y, Wyon MA. Physiological fitness and professional classical ballet performance: a brief review. J Strength Cond Res 2009;23(9): 2732–40.
11. Rodrigues-Krause J, Dos Santos Cunha G, Alberton CL, et al. Oxygen consumption and heart rate responses to isolated ballet exercise sets. J Dance Med Sci 2014;18(3):99–105.
12. Angioi M, Metsios GS, Metsios G, et al. Fitness in contemporary dance: a systematic review. Int J Sports Med 2009;30(7):475–84.
13. Rafferty S. Considerations for integrating fitness into dance training. J Dance Med Sci 2010;14(2):45–9.
14. Schantz PG, Astrand PO. Physiological characteristics of classical ballet. Med Sci Sports Exerc 1984;16(5):472–6.
15. Guarina L. Is dance a sport?: a twenty-first-century debate. J Dance Educ 2015; 15:77–80.
16. Kenny SJ, Palacios-Derflingher L, Whittaker JL, et al. The influence of injury definition on injury burden in preprofessional ballet and contemporary dancers. J Orthop Sports Phys Ther 2018;48(3):185–93.
17. Jacobs CL, Hincapié CA, Cassidy JD. Musculoskeletal injuries and pain in dancers: a systematic review update. J Dance Med Sci 2012;16(2):74–84.
18. Jacobs CL, Cassidy JD, Côté P, et al. Musculoskeletal injury in professional dancers: prevalence and associated factors: an international cross-sectional study. Clin J Sport Med 2017;27(2):153–60.
19. Roberts KJ, Nelson NG, McKenzie L. Dance-related injuries in children and adolescents treated in US emergency departments in 1991-2007. J Phys Act Health 2013;10(2):143–50.

20. Leanderson C, Leanderson J, Wykman A, et al. Musculoskeletal injuries in young ballet dancers. Knee Surg Sports Traumatol Arthrosc 2011;19(9):1531–5.
21. Russell JA. Preventing dance injuries: current perspectives. Open Access J Sports Med 2013;4:199–210.
22. Malkogeorgos A, Mavrovouniotis F, Zaggelidis G, et al. Common dance related musculoskeletal injuries. J Phys Educ Sport 2011;11(3):259–66.
23. Bronner S, McBride C, Gill A. Musculoskeletal injuries in professional modern dancers: a prospective cohort study of 15 years. J Sports Sci 2018;36(16): 1880–8.
24. Allen N, Nevill AM, Brooks JH, et al. The effect of a comprehensive injury audit program on injury incidence in ballet: a 3-year prospective study. Clin J Sport Med 2013;23(5):373–8.
25. Nilsson C, Leanderson J, Wykman A, et al. The injury panorama in a Swedish professional ballet company. Knee Surg Sports Traumatol Arthrosc 2001;9(4):242–6.
26. Ramkumar PN, Farber J, Arnouk J, et al. Injuries in a professional ballet dance company: a 10-year retrospective study. J Dance Med Sci 2016;20(1):30–7.
27. Vassallo AJ, Trevor BL, Mota L, et al. Injury rates and characteristics in recreational, elite student and professional dancers: a systematic review. J Sports Sci 2019;37(10):1113–22.
28. Beasley MA, Stracciolini A, Tyson KD, et al. Knee injury patterns in young Irish dancers. Med Probl Perform Art 2014;29(2):70–3.
29. Stein CJ, Tyson KD, Johnson VM, et al. Injuries in Irish dance. J Dance Med Sci 2013;17(4):159–64.
30. Kauther MD, Wedemeyer C, Wegner A, et al. Breakdance injuries and overuse syndromes in amateurs and professionals. Am J Sports Med 2009;37(4): 797–802.
31. Gamboa JM, Roberts LA, Maring J, et al. Injury patterns in elite preprofessional ballet dancers and the utility of screening programs to identify risk characteristics. J Orthop Sports Phys Ther 2008;38(3):126–36.
32. Ojofeitimi S, Bronner S. Injuries in a modern dance company effect of comprehensive management on injury incidence and cost. J Dance Med Sci 2011; 15(3):116–22.
33. Lee L, Reid D, Cadwell J, et al. Injury incidence, dance exposure and the use of the movement competency screen (MCS) to identify variables associated with injury in full-time pre-professional dancers. Int J Sports Phys Ther 2017;12(3): 352–70.
34. Ekegren CL, Quested R, Brodrick A. Injuries in pre-professional ballet dancers: incidence, characteristics and consequences. J Sci Med Sport 2014;17(3): 271–5.
35. Allen N, Wyon M. Dance medicine: artist or athlete? SportEx Medicine 2008; 35:6–9.
36. Heyward VH. Advanced fitness assessment and exercise prescription. 6th edition. Champaign (IL): Human Kinetics; 2010.
37. Gamble P. Implications and applications of training specificity for coaches and athletes. Strength Cond J 2006;28(3):54–8.
38. Storm JM, Wolman R, Bakker EWP, et al. The relationship between range of motion and injuries in adolescent dancers and sportspersons: a systematic review. Front Psychol 2018;9:287.
39. McCormack MC, Bird H, de Medici A, et al. The physical attributes most required in professional ballet: a Delphi study. Sports Med Int Open 2019;3(1):E1–5.

40. Bennell K, Khan KM, Matthews B, et al. Hip and ankle range of motion and hip muscle strength in young female ballet dancers and controls. Br J Sports Med 1999;33(5):340–6.
41. Kraemer W, McNerney J, Pallay R, et al. The team physician and conditioning of athletes for sports: a consensus statement. Med Sci Sports Exerc 2001;33(10): 1789–93.
42. Liederbach M, Richardson M, Rodriguez M, et al. Jump exposures in the dance training environment: a measure of ergonomic demand. J Athl Train 2006;41:S85.
43. Wyon M. Preparing to perform: periodization and dance. J Dance Med Sci 2010; 14(2):67–72.
44. Bronner S, Ojofeitimi S, Lora JB, et al. A preseason cardiorespiratory profile of dancers in nine professional ballet and modern companies. J Dance Med Sci 2014;18(2):74–85.
45. Bailey M. Raising the barre: how science is saving ballet dancers. 2018. Available at: https://www.theguardian.com/stage/2018/jul/15/raising-the-barre-how-science-is-saving-ballet-dancers. Accessed April 6, 2020.
46. Fitness and Conditioning. The Australian Ballet School. Available at: https://www.australianballetschool.com.au/pages/fitness-and-conditioning. Accessed April 30,2020.
47. Guardian T. Batsheva Dance Company: 'It's about making the body listen." In. Youtube 2013. Available at: https://youtu.be/gRky99sO-og. Accessed April 6, 2020.
48. Company BD. Echad Mi Yodea by Ohad Narahin performed by Batsheva - the Young Ensemble. In. Youtube 2016. Available at: https://www.youtube.com/watch?v=7v6tY_u-Mls.
49. Tabata I, Nishimura K, Kouzaki M, et al. Effects of moderate-intensity endurance and high-intensity intermittent training on anaerobic capacity and VO2max. Med Sci Sports Exerc 1996;28(10):1327–30.
50. Murach K, Bagley J. Less is more: the physiological basis for tapering in endurance, strength, and power athletes. Sports 2015;3:209–18.
51. Faulkner E, Blackmon A. Development of a choreography-specific conditioning program to help prepare classical dancers for contemporary performances Paper presented at: International Association for Dance Medicine and Science 2018. Helsinki, October 25-28, 2018.

Supplemental Training in Dance: A Systematic Review

Jatin P. Ambegaonkar, PhD, ATC, OT, CSCS, FIADMS[a],*,
Lillian Chong, BS, ACSM-EP[b], Pranjal Joshi, MS[b]

KEYWORDS

- Cross-training • Pathology • Performing artists • Performance • Aesthetics

KEY POINTS

- The effects of supplemental training in dancers have been examined in smaller studies with small samples and in mostly collegiate female dancers.
- Studies examining supplemental training in dancers have generally low rigor, low level of evidence, and low strength of recommendations.
- Supplemental training programs that include multiple exercises, last around 1 hour per session, and are implemented 2 to 3 times per week for around 8 weeks seem to enhance dancers' performance.
- Only limited evidence exists for using supplemental training to reduce dancers' low back pain and injury risk.
- Overall, practitioners can use review findings to advocate supplemental training inclusion in dancers' practice regimens to provide performance enhancement and injury risk reduction.

INTRODUCTION

Dancing, like athletics, is a rigorous physical activity.[1-4] Therefore, dancers require physical fitness including strength, speed, power, agility, cardiovascular endurance, flexibility, coordination, and balance to meet performance demands.[5] However, unlike athletics, dancing also requires participants to perform aesthetically pleasing movements without getting injured.[1,4,6,7] Because of these high mental and physical demands, dancers have an increased risk of injury.[8-10] Dancers experience cumulative injury incidences ranging from 17% to 94%[8,10,11] and injury prevalence of 4.4

Conflict of interest: None.
Funding: None.
[a] Sports Medicine Assessment Research and Testing (SMART) Laboratory, George Mason University, 201-F, K Johnson Hall, MSN 4E5, 10890 George Mason Circle, Manassas, VA 20110, USA;
[b] Sports Medicine Assessment Research and Testing (SMART) Laboratory, George Mason University, MSN 4E5, 10890 George Mason Circle, Manassas, VA 20110, USA
* Corresponding author.
E-mail address: jambegao@gmu.edu

injuries/1000 hours during a single season, which is higher than in some prior reports in athletes.[8,12–16] Overall, dance is a unique combination of art and sport that requires athletic activity with a lack of specificity and periodicity in training, movement in extreme ranges of motion, artistic expression, and musicality.[8,17–20]

Previous investigators have suggested that dance training alone may not be able to provide adequate physical fitness,[3,21,22] and have recommended additional training programs (synonymous with supplemental or cross-training in this article) to enhance performance and/or reduce injury risk in dancers.[2,23–28] Although athletes often take part in supplemental training programs,[2–4,29] fewer studies have examined these training programs in dancers.

Little published research exists detailing the forms, dosage, and timing of these training programs in dancers. Moreover, how taking part in supplemental training affects dancers' performance and injury risk also remains unclear. This lack of information may make it difficult for dancers, educators, clinicians, and practitioners working with dancers and performing artists to devise training programs to enhance dancers' performance and reduce their injury risk.[30,31] This lack of information may also unintentionally promote the previously described disproportionate focus on skill acquisition rather than fitness that is prevalent in dance.[2,30,31]

Overall, despite the high physical rigors and injury rates in dance, and health care providers often caring for dancers, what types of supplemental training have been used in dancers is uncertain. How these training methods affect their performance or injury risk also remains unclear. Therefore, this article examines (1) types of supplemental training used by dancers, and (2) effects of supplemental training on performance and injury risk in dancers.

METHODOLOGY
Protocol and Registration

The authors registered this review on the Center for Reviews and Dissemination International Prospective Register of Systematic Reviews register (CRD42020172294). We conducted the review according to the Preferred Reporting Items for Systematic review and Meta-Analyses (PRISMA) guidelines.[32]

Search Methods

Nine databases (EBSCO Host, Web of Science, ProQuest Performing Arts, CINAHL Plus, SPORTDiscus, ERIC, PubMed, Cochrane Library, and Education Research Complete) were systematically searched for studies using the search terms shown in **Table 1** through March 1 2020. Titles and abstracts were screened for inclusion based on eligibility criteria. Inclusion and exclusion criteria are shown in **Table 2**.

Scoring Methods

Two independent reviewers assessed the methodological quality of the studies using the modified Downs and Black[33] (mDB) criteria, yielding a score out of 28 possible points (0%–100%). This valid and reliable tool has been classified to examine the methodological rigor of both randomized and nonrandomized studies (ie, observational, epidemiologic).[33] Studies scoring less than 60% were deemed low quality, between 60% and 74.9% indicates moderate quality, and greater than or equal to 75% suggests high quality of methodological rigor.[33]

The strength of recommendations was determined using the Strength of Recommendation Taxonomy (SORT) tool, which includes A, B, and C grades.[34] Grade A is considered consistent, good-quality patient-oriented evidence.[34] Grade B

Table 1
Keywords and search terms used in the systematic review of supplemental training and dance

Step	Search Terms	Boolean Operator	EBSCO Host	Web of Science	ProQuest Performing Arts	CINAHL Plus	SPORTDiscus	ERIC	PubMed	Cochrane Library	Education Research Complete
1	Dance*	—	27,591	56,202	16,864	2881	11,099	5745	12,450	1613	7866
2	Train*	—	481,568	993,805	12,762	137,865	81,760	78,709	550,490	103,963	183,234
3	Supplement*	—	109,057	488,291	4002	53,709	36,957	6304	309,025	87,880	12,087
4	Exercis*	—	278,734	475,468	7664	106,198	115,611	15,940	349,229	98,954	40,985
5	Cross Train*	—	3774	51,096	4635	1082	700	1134	519	8289	858
6	Fitness	—	69,874	143,844	1056	15,359	38,429	3149	85,648	11,195	12,937
7	2, 3, 4, 5, 6	OR	800,139	1,956,897	18,283	276,737	191,500	99,909	1,169,221	245,149	231,993
8	1, 7	AND	11,145	4048	9181	969	5581	1872	2766	888	2723
9	8	NOT Animal	11,102	3983	7257	964	5566	1866	2601	773	2706
10	Injur*	—	293,714	961,542	3191	206,129	64,319	3831	950,204	61,609	19,435
11	8, 9, 10	AND	1004	410	961	271	527	80	439	65	126

* denotes wildcard search term.

Table 2
Inclusion and exclusion criteria used in the systematic review of supplemental training and dance

Inclusion Criteria	Exclusion Criteria
Studies examining effects of supplemental training in dancers	Studies that included only retired dancers
Participants in 1 or more groups were described as current dancers	Case studies, conference proceedings, or review articles
Studies published in English	Studies that limited participants to those with chronic diseases (eg, asthma)
Studies published in peer-reviewed journals	Studies that described only the development of supplemental training protocol

recommendations are inconsistent, limited-quality patient-oriented evidence.[34] Grade C is considered consensus or case series for studies of diagnosis, treatment, prevention, or screening.[34]

Studies were evaluated for evidence level based on the Oxford Centre for Evidence-Based Medicine Levels of Evidence (LOE) tool. This tool ranks research from level 1 to level 5, with level 1 being ranked as the highest evidence.[35] Any disagreement was resolved by discussion, and a third reviewer was available when consensus could not be reached.

The following data were extracted from the included studies: study design, sample size, participant characteristics (age, sex, level of dancer, type of dance), types and dosage (per session, per week, total) of supplemental training, outcome measures used to examine effects of supplemental training, and effects of supplemental training.

SYNTHESIS
Included Studies

The initial search retrieved 2540 articles (**Fig. 1**). Following the initial screening, 885 articles were discarded by removing abstracts, duplicates, or reviews. Thereafter, 1607 articles were discarded after reviewing either their titles and/or abstracts. Of the 48 remaining articles, 37 were discarded after reviewing the full text, leaving 11 studies that met the final eligibility criteria and initial complete review. After reviewing these full-text articles, 3 additional articles were identified from the back references that met eligibility criteria, resulting in 14 final included articles. A meta-analysis of the supplemental training programs could not be conducted because of the heterogeneity of dance genres, methods, and outcome measures.

Study Design and Participants Characteristics

Study design
Of the 14 studies, only 3[4,36,37] used some form of a randomized controlled trial study design, whereas the others used convenience or nonrandom cohort samples for case-control[7,28,29,38–40] or single-group pre-post study design.[6,30,41–43] Although 8 out of 14 studies had some control group,[4,7,28,29,36,38–40] others used the same dancers in a within-subjects repeated-measures design.[6,30,37,41–43]

Participants
All 14 studies (total participants = 387) included women (n = 376), with only 2 studies[36,39] examining both sexes (total men, n = 11), with (mean ± standard deviation

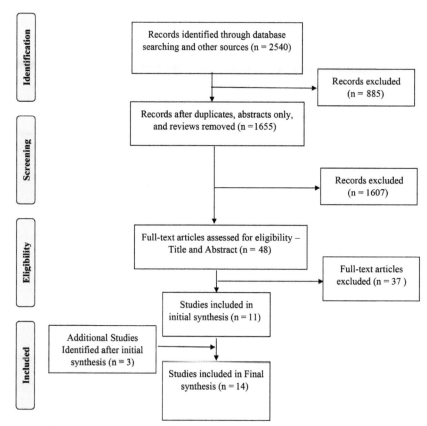

Fig. 1. Included studies in the systematic review of supplemental training and dance.

[SD]) 29.4 ± 18.9 participants/study (range, 6–62 dancers). The participants were young (20.7 + 4.0 years; range: 13–27 years).

Dancer levels and genres

Most of the studies (10 of 14) examined collegiate dancers,[4,7,29,36,38–43] whereas 3 studies were conducted with professional dancers,[4,28,37] and 1 each examined adolescent[30] and preprofessional dancers.[6] The dance genres included mixed (n = 7),[7,30,36,38,40,42,43] modern/contemporary (n = 4),[4,37,39] and ballet (n = 4),[6,28,29,39,41] with 1 study examining hip-hop dancers[6] and 1 examining competitive collegiate dancers.[43] Note that the total numbers of dancer levels and genres are more than the total number of included studies because several studies included dancers across multiple levels and genres (**Table 3**).

Types and Dosage of Supplemental Training

Types

There was substantial variability in the types and dosages of training programs. Note that the types of training are more than the total number of included studies because several studies included multiple types across multiple levels and genres. The most common types of supplemental training included strength (synonymous with resistance and weight in the current review; n = 8),[4,6,7,28–30,36,40] core stability training

Table 3
Summary of study demographics included in the systematic review of supplemental training and dance

	Study	Training Level	Mean Age (y)	Sex	Dance Genre	Female (n)	Male (n)	Total (N)
1	Angioi et al,[4] 2012	14 collegiate and 10 professional	27	24 F	Contemporary	24	0	24
2	Brown et al,[7] 2007	18 collegiate	19.7	18 F	Mixed	18	0	18
3	Dowse et al,[30] 2017	12 adolescent	14.2	12 F	Mixed	12	0	12
4	Grossman & Wilmerding,[38] 2000	16 collegiate	NR	16 F	Mixed	16	0	16
5	Kalaycioglu et al,[41] 2020	24 collegiate	21.4	NR	Ballet and modern	24	0	24
6	Karim et al,[37] 2019	59 professional	25.78	59 F	Contemporary	59	0	59
7	Koutedakis et al,[39] 2007	32 collegiate	19.75	27 F/5 M	Contemporary and ballet	27	5	32
8	Koutedakis et al,[28] 2004	22 professional	25	22 F	Ballet	22	0	22
9	Kovácsné et al,[6] 2016	62 preprofessional	13.2	NR	Ballet and hip-hop	62	0	62
10	Pata et al,[42] 2014	6 collegiate	NR	6 F	Mixed	6	0	6
11	Roussel et al,[36] 2014	44 collegiate	19.75	38 F/6 M	Mixed	38	6	44
12	Stalder et al,[29] 1990	14 collegiate	21.85	14 F	Ballet	14	0	14
13	Stošić et al,[40] 2019	54 collegiate	NR	54 F	Mixed	54	0	54
14	Watson et al,[43] 2017	24 collegiate	19.7	24 F	Mixed, competitive collegiate	24	0	24

Abbreviations: F, female; M, male; NR, not reported.
Data from Refs.[4,6,7,28–30,36–43]

(n = 3),[6,41,43] aerobic (n = 2),[36,39] plyometrics (n = 2),[7,40] whole-body vibration (n = 2),[4,37] and other forms of site-specific conditioning training (eg, range of motion, motor control, proprioception). Some researchers asked dancers to perform a single exercise (eg, a modified leg raise)[38] or asked participants to perform a single motion (eg, demi plié) during whole-body vibration training,[37] whereas most of the other researchers used multimodal, combined, or multiple joint activities.

Dosage

The dosage of training also varied widely across the studies. When considering training time per session, Karim and colleagues[37] used a 75-second session of whole-body vibration, whereas Roussel and colleagues[36] had training sessions lasting 150 minutes. The number of times per week that researchers implemented training also varied, with most researchers providing interventions 2 to 3[4,7,28–30,38–41,43] times per week and others, such as Pata and colleagues,[42] performing interventions for 10 consecutive days. To collate these weekly variations, we converted and averaged training dosage as a function of a week (eg, 1 day = one-seventh of a week or 0.14 week; 10 days = 1.4 weeks). The total program durations ranged from a single session[37] to a 4-month period.[36] Overall, the training programs were implemented for an average of 54.9 ± 42.2 min/session, 2.4 ± 0.9 times per week for 8.3 ± 4.3 weeks. Consistent information about timing of program implementation across a dance season was not found (**Table 4**).

Outcome Measures Used to Examine Effects of Supplemental Training

Heterogeneity existed in outcome measures to examine effects of supplemental training, with researchers using almost 50 different outcome measures. To organize these disparate measures, we created 3 broad categories: (1) functional fitness, not just dance specific (eg, aerobic capacity, power, endurance, balance), (2) discrete (eg, anthropometrics, injury), and (3) dance specific (eg, aesthetic performance, dance competence). Given that multiple studies included several outcome measures, the total numbers of outcome measures were more than the total numbers of studies.

Specifically, in the functional fitness category, the most common differing types of outcome measures were muscle power (n = 10)[4,7,28–30,36,37,40,41,43]; balance, proprioception, and coordination (n = 9)[6,30,37,40,41,43]; strength (n = 7)[6,7,29,30,39,41,43]; endurance (n = 4)[4,43]; and aerobic capacity (n = 3).[4,36,39] Several researchers examined different anthropometrics (n = 7),[28,29,38,39,41] with others examining habitual posture (n = 1),[6] pain (n = 2),[6,36] injury (n = 1),[36] habitual physical activity (n = 1),[36] and health-related quality of life (n = 1).[36] Interestingly, only 57.4% of the studies (8 of 14)[4,7,29,30,36,39,42,43] examined dance-specific activity or movement including dance competence or aesthetics in some form. These dance-specific activities were rated using a combination of subjective ratings, scores, and scales.

Effects of Supplemental Training

In general, when examining performance, supplemental training seemed to enhance performance across a variety of outcome measures (**Table 5**). However, when considering pain or injury, only 2 groups[6,36] reported that dancers reported fewer low back injuries and/or less pain after taking part in a physical conditioning program compared with a health promotion program that did not include any training or exercise program.

Methodological Rigor and Scoring

The mean mDB scores were 59.8 ± 7.5% (16.8 ± 1.6) indicating overall low methodological rigor (**Table 6**). Half the studies (7 of 14) were scored less than 60% (low

Table 4
Summary of participant groups and types and dosage of supplemental training in dance

Study	Participants (n/Group)	Supplemental Training Type	Training Time/Session (min)	Training Times/wk	Total Training Duration (wk)
Angioi et al,[4] 2012	12 E/12 C	Strength training and whole body vibration	60	2	6
Brown et al,[7] 2007	6 plyometrics/ 6 strength/6 C	Plyometrics and strength training	37.5	2	6
Dowse et al,[30] 2017	12 E	Strength training	52.5	2	9
Grossman & Wilmerding,[38] 2000	8 E/8 C	Site-specific conditioning	5	2.5	6
Kalaycioglu et al,[41] 2020	24 E	Core stability training	52.5	3	8
Karim et al,[37] 2019	29 E/30 C	Whole-body vibration	1.25	0	0.14
Koutedakis et al,[39] 2007	19 E/13 C	Aerobic and strength training	50	3	12
Koutedakis et al,[28] 2004	12 E/10 C	Strength training	50	3	12
Kovácsné et al,[5] 2016	62 E	Core stability training	NR	NR	12
Pata et al,[42] 2014	6 E	Site-specific conditioning	NR	NR	1.4
Roussel et al,[36] 2014	23 E/21 C	Aerobic and strength training	150	NR	16
Stalder et al,[29] 1990	7 E/7 C	Strength training	NR	3	9
Stošić et al,[40] 2019	27 E/27 C	Strength training and plyometrics	90	3	10
Watson et al,[43] 2017	24 E	Core Stability training	NR	3	9

Abbreviations: C, control; E, experimental.
Data from Refs.[4,6,7,28–30,36–40,42,43]

Table 5
Outcome measures used to examine effects of supplemental training and dance

Category	Outcome Measures	Study	Specific Measure (Measurement Units)	Improvements
Functional fitness	Muscular power	Angioi et al,[4] 2012	Vertical Jump (cm)	Yes
		Brown et al,[7] 2007	Wingate Anaerobic Power Test: peak and mean power (W), vertical jump (cm) standing and moving (cm)	Yes
		Dowse et al,[30] 2017	Squat jump peak power (W) and relative peak power (W/kg), countermovement jump peak power (W) and relative peak power (W/kg), single-leg counter movement jump peak power (W), eccentric utilization ratio, limb power symmetry ratio	Yes
		Kalaycioglu et al,[41] 2020	Vertical jump test (cm), dominant and nondominant	Yes[a]
		Karim et al,[37] 2019	Countermovement jumps: sautés (cm)	No
		Koutedakis et al,[28] 2004	Hamstring and quadriceps muscle torque (N.m)	Yes
		Stalder et al,[29] 1990	Anaerobic power using stair running test (kg/m/s)	Yes
		Roussel et al,[36] 2014	Standing broad jump (m)	No
		Stosić et al,[40] 2019	Squat jump and countermovement jump (measurement units NR)	Yes
	Muscular strength	Watson et al,[43] 2017	Single-leg Hop Test (% normalized for leg length)	Yes
		Brown et al,[7] 2007	Strength (kg) of leg press, knee curl, and knee extension	Yes
		Dowse et al,[30] 2017	Isometric midthigh pull (N)	Yes
		Kalaycioglu et al,[41] 2020	Hip flexor/extensor isokinetics, peak torques (Nm/kg), total work (j)	No
		Koutedakis et al,[39] 2007	Bilateral isometric knee extensor strength (kg)	Yes
		Kovácsné et al,[6] 2016	Static strength of core muscles (score when maintaining push-up for 120 s)	Yes
		Stalder et al,[29] 1990	Isometric strength knee extensor strength, ankle plantar and dorsiflexion (kg)	Yes
	Muscular endurance	Watson et al,[43] 2017	Hip abductor strength (kg)	Yes
		Angioi et al,[4] 2012	Press-ups (times/min)	Yes
		Angioi et al,[4] 2012	Jumping for 2-min with metronome	Yes
		Watson et al,[43] 2017	Back extensor, abdominal, side bridge core endurance tests (s)	Yes
		Watson et al,[43] 2017	Single-leg heel raise (repetitions)	No

(continued on next page)

Table 5
(continued)

Category	Outcome Measures	Study	Specific Measure (Measurement Units)	Improvements
	Aerobic capacity	Angioi et al,[4] 2012	Dance Aerobic Fitness Test, aerobic heart rate (beats/min) at 46 mL/kg/min)	Yes
		Koutedakis et al,[39] 2007	VO_{2max} (mL/kg/min)	Yes
		Roussel et al,[36] 2014	Aerobic capacity VO_{2max} (mL/kg) and relative VO_{2Max} (mL/kg/min), peak ventilation (L/min), heart rate (beats/min), systolic and diastolic blood pressure (mm Hg), maximal workload (W), Borg Rate of Perceived Exertion using electronically braked bicycle ergometer	No
	Balance, proprioception, coordination	Dowse et al,[30] 2017	Dynamic balance using Biodex Balance System, Overall Stability Index, Anterior-Posterior Stability Index, Medial-lateral Stability Index	Yes [a]
		Kalaycioglu et al,[41] 2020	Y Balance Test (cm)	Yes [a]
		Kalaycioglu et al,[41] 2020	Proprioception and coordination using active reproduction of joint position (cm)	No
		Kalaycioglu et al,[41] 2020	Coordination using Swiss ball and stability trainer with eyes open and closed	Yes
		Karim et al,[37] 2019	Star Excursion Balance Test (cm), Balance Error Scoring System (errors)	No
		Kovácsné et al,[6] 2016	Lumbar motor control ability using Leg-lowering Test (maintain 45 mm Hg from 40 mm Hg)	Yes
		Stošić et al,[40] 2019	Coordination using 6 tests: Side Steps, Forward Steps Twirling Baton, Skipping Rope, Turning in 6 Squares, Hand-foot Drumming, Agility with Baton (score)	Yes [a]
		Watson et al,[43] 2017	Single-leg balance in passé relevé (s)	Yes [a]
		Watson et al,[43] 2017	Star Excursion Balance Test (% normalized for leg length)	Yes [a]

Category	Subcategory	Reference	Description	Support
Discrete tests		Grossman & Wilmerding,[38] 2000	Height of gesture leg (cm) extension in à la seconde	Yes
	Anthropometrics	Kalaycioglu et al,[41] 2020	Flexibility using Sit and Reach Test (cm)	No
		Koutedakis et al,[28] 2004	Body mass (kg), sum of skinfolds (mm), fat-free mass (kg), thigh circumference (cm)	Yes [a]
		Koutedakis et al,[39] 2007	Flexibility using straight right leg raise (degrees)	Yes [a]
		Koutedakis et al,[39] 2007	Sum of 4 skinfolds (mm)	No
		Stalder et al,[29] 1990	Thigh and calf circumference (cm)	No
		Stalder et al,[29] 1990	Anterior, posterior, lateral leg flexion, ankle plantar and dorsiflexion (degrees)	Yes[a]
	Posture	Kovácsné et al,[6] 2016	Habitual Posture Score change (1 front, 2 side-view photographs)	Yes
	Pain	Kovácsné et al,[6] 2016	Intensity of low back pain using visual analog scale (0–100)	Yes
	Injury	Roussel et al,[36] 2014	Self-reported 12-mo recall of symptoms of pain or discomfort in neck, upper back, low back, hips/thighs, knees, ankle/feet. Injuries included if time loss only (cumulative incidence proportions, injury incidence rate/1000 h of dance)	Yes [a]
	Physical activity	Roussel et al,[36] 2014	Baecke Habitual Physical Activity Questionnaire (work, sports, nonsports)	No
	Health-related quality of life	Roussel et al,[36] 2014	Short Form 36	No
Dance specific	Aesthetic competence/dance	Angioi et al,[4] 2012	Contemporary Dance Aesthetic Competence Test (score)	Yes
		Brown et al,[7] 2007	Subjective evaluation: ballon, jump height, feet pointing, overall ability	Yes[a]
	performance qualitative ratings	Dowse et al,[30] 2017	Subjective evaluation of dance performance, control, spatial skills, accuracy, technique, dynamics, and overall performance (score to 60)	Yes
		Koutedakis et al,[39] 2007	Custom designed dance test that included parallel sideways jumps (score)	Yes
		Stalder et al,[29] 1990	Ratings of dance-specific muscle endurance when performing sauté changement, petit allegro combination (subjectively scored by instructors)	Yes [a]
	Dance-specific quantitative scores	Roussel et al,[36] 2014	Dance Functional Outcome Scale	No
		Pata et al,[42] 2014	Total active turnout (degrees)	Yes
		Watson et al,[43] 2017	Dance performance pirouettes (maximum revolutions)	Yes

[a] Only partial support.
Data from Refs.[4,6,7,28–30,36,38–43]

Table 6
Methodological quality of included studies in the systematic review of supplemental training and dance

Study	mDB Scores	mDB (%)	LOE
Angioi et al,[4] 2012	16	57.1	2
Brown et al,[7] 2007	18	64.3	3
Dowse et al,[30] 2017	15	53.6	3
Grossman & Wilmerding,[38] 2000	18	64.3	4
Kalaycioglu et al,[41] 2020	16	57.1	3
Karim et al,[37] 2019	19	67.9	2
Koutedakis et al,[39] 2007	19	67.9	3
Koutedakis et al,[28] 2004	15	53.6	3
Kovácsné et al,[6] 2016	15	53.6	3
Pata et al,[42] 2014	17	60.7	4
Roussel et al,[36] 2014	19	67.9	2
Stalder et al,[29] 1990	15	53.6	3
Stošić et al,[40] 2019	16	57.1	3
Watson et al,[43] 2017	17	60.7	3

mDB criteria provide a score of 0 to 28, or 0% to 100%: less than 60%, low quality; 60% to 74.9%, moderate quality; and greater than or equal to 75%, high quality of methodological rigor. LOE based on Oxford Centre for Evidence-based Medicine 2011 Levels of Evidence tool (see Table 1).
    Data from Refs.[4,6,7,28–30,36–40,42,43]

quality)[4,6,28–30,40,41] and none of the studies scored more than 75% (high quality) in methodological rigor. The 14 studies ranged in B to C strength of recommendations, supporting supplemental training use to improve performance, and level C evidence for supporting supplemental training use in reducing low back pain and injury. According to the Oxford grading level, most studies had level 3 LOE.

DISCUSSION
Primary Findings

In general, the studies in the current systematic review had small sample sizes and examined mostly collegiate women. The supplemental training programs were around 1 hour long, 2 to 3 times per week, and were implemented for around 8 weeks. Researchers examined the effects of supplemental training using either discrete tests or fitness assessments not specific to dance, with only a few studying specific dance performance or aesthetics. The studies had generally low to moderate methodological rigor and weak strength of recommendation.

Study Design and Participant Characteristics

Most studies had small sample sizes (range, 6–62). In contrast, several research groups have examined training in much larger sample sizes in sports medicine and athletics settings.[15,44–46] Given that the average number of participants in the current review was less than 30, we can only make limited recommendations about associations between training and performance or injury risk. Also, because of the use of convenience samples and the lack of randomization or matching in most studies, selection bias was a likely confounder in the current review. We also found a lack of consistency of control/comparison groups versus experimental groups across the studies. Whether using nondancer controls and using the same group measures repeatedly provides appropriate information to make valid recommendations about dancers remains unclear, especially given that dancers have been noted to be weaker than other physically active populations.[47–49]

Similar to other systematic reviews of dancers,[3,5,10,11,25,50] we found a larger number of women as participants than men. However, the glaring discrepancy in numbers of women versus men (almost 400 women vs 11 men) is a matter of concern, especially given that male dancers have been reported to have rigorous physical demands, and even higher upper body injury rates than female dancers.[10,25] The current findings thus suggest a gap in the current literature about the effects of supplemental training in male dancers and is a recommended area for future work.

Although the finding that most participants across the studies were collegiate dance students is likely in part a result of sample of convenience issue mentioned earlier, student dancers have been suggested to be the largest percentage of dancers.[51] Alternatively, despite the high demands[9,21,52,53] and work volumes[9] in professional dance, fewer studies have examined this elite group. Understanding the effects of supplemental training on performance and injury risk is especially important at this level, given that professional dancers' livelihoods and careers depend on being able to perform well and stay healthy. Although the current findings indicate that adding supplemental training may be beneficial for dancers, clarifying the optimal volumes of supplemental training is needed, given that fatigue and overwork is a known concern for professional dancers.[21,54]

As expected, the most frequent dance styles included were mixed, modern, and ballet. However, other forms of dance (eg, Irish, Indian classical, hip-hop, breaking, theatrical)[23,54–60] have differing demands and are becoming increasingly popular. In a recent systematic review and meta-analysis,[5] researchers found that dance-specific positions could predict injury, and noted that movements were genre specific (in this case, ballet), and thus not likely relevant to other dance genres. Combining our findings with these observations suggests a need for research work across dance genres to examine the prevalence and types of supplemental training performed by dancers taking part in other genres. Practitioners also should examine whether these programs affect dancers of different genres and levels differently.

Types and Dosage of Supplemental Training

In general, the supplemental training program dosage was 1 hour, 2 to 3 times per week for around 8 weeks, with a wide variety of supplemental training methods. The protocols varied from single motions[38] to comprehensive multimodal programs.[36] In general, longer and more frequent training resulted in greater adaptions. These findings are in agreement with prior systematic reviews and meta-analyses, where investigators[61,62] noted that plyometric training improved performance in female athletes regardless of age, type of sport, and competition level, and that longer training durations provided larger improvements.

As in athletics, dancers also have different cycles with differing demands (eg, off-season, preseason, in-season).[22] The demands on the dancers' bodies and the goals vary (eg, increase strength during the off-season, maintain skill and performance during the in-season) during these macrocycles.[22] Dancers' performance and injury risk should also consequently vary across the season. Therefore, the effects of a supplemental training program implemented in-season may differ from implementation off-season, and is an area of needed investigation.

In the current review, consistent information about timing of supplemental training across a dance season was not found. Other investigators have also noted the need for considering timing of training. For example, Roussel and colleagues[36] proposed that researchers should explore how additional training may be organized around the dancers' daily schedules. Likewise, Koutedakis and Sharp[28] advocated more research on the effects of systematic off-studio physical fitness training on dancer performance. Combining all these opinions, the authors recommend that researchers should consider the time in the dancers' season when they implement supplemental training and match the program goals with performance demands.

We also could not find consistency in who designed and/or delivered these programs (ie, on-site athletic trainers, physical therapists, strength and conditioning coaches, exercise physiologists, dancers, and so forth). We also noted inconsistencies in whether the programs were supervised or performed by dancers themselves without supervision of a trained instructor. Given that several programs were designed to progressively load the body and cause performance enhancements,[41] if dancers perform these programs incorrectly there may be negative outcomes. The least problematic outcome being that the programs are ineffective, with the most problematic being that the programs may cause injury and harm the dancer. Although we could not draw firm conclusions from the limited available data, anecdotally we recommended that supplemental training programs should be implemented by a professional trained in dance medicine and familiar with the demands of the dancer's season. On the whole, more research is required to devise dancer-specific programs that are easy to implement inside and outside studio settings.

Outcome Measures Used to Examine Effects of Supplemental Training

Western dance is often characterized by short bursts of explosive activity that require anaerobic power and strength to perform leaps and jumps.[7,30,40] Dancers also need to have superior balance, coordination, and proprioception to maintain aesthetics during performance.[4,24,40,63] Thus, dancers require strength, speed, power, agility, cardiovascular endurance, flexibility, coordination and balance, and visually pleasing aesthetics.[4,6,7,48] Given this wide range of demands, it was interesting to note that supplemental training effects were examined using fitness assessments that were not always dance specific, with fewer researchers examining dance aesthetics or competence. These findings are understandable given the subjective nature of grading dance aesthetics, but highlight the challenges of determining the success of physical fitness supplemental training in dance. Overall, the authors agree with Kalaycioglu and colleagues,[41] who suggested that future research should include functional assessments and field tests and identify a need to customize these to be dance-studio friendly and low tech to promote user-friendliness for teachers, choreographers, and performers.

Intriguingly, despite several prior investigators suggesting use of training to decrease injury risk in dancers,[44,45,64] we found only 2 studies[6,36] examining the effects of supplemental training on disorder or injury. Roussel and colleagues[36] found that, although 4 months of training did not alter any specific fitness parameters, it did reduce dancers' complaints of self-reported 12-month recall of low back pain. Kovácsné and colleagues[6] found that dancers reported decreased low back pain intensity after taking part in the exercise program.

Roussel and colleagues[36] also commented that they did not have a true control group, and that they recorded information for only 4 months. None of the other studies examined injury or performed long-term follow-up assessments after their immediate postintervention assessments. Hence, we do not know whether dancers continued to perform supplemental training, or whether there were any lasting effects of the supplemental training programs on dancers' performance or injury risk. Taken as a whole, this lack of information represents a substantial gap in the field. Thus, in agreement with Roussel and colleagues,[36] we identify a need for multicenter and longitudinal prospective research to examine associations between injury risk and supplemental training in dancers.

Effects of Supplemental Training

In general, most researchers found that supplemental training improved performance, and researchers in a couple of studies noted reduced low back pain and injury. The performance measures ranged from general fitness measures to dance-specific motions and aesthetics. One of the most interesting observations was that none of the studies examined any psychological or mental outcome measures. In a recent systematic review of health-related quality-of-life measures used in dance, the investigators reported that, although 8 different measures were used to examine dancers' health-related quality of life, all measures examined some construct of mental health. This finding is important considering the mental aspect of dance.[65] Hence researchers need to compare different forms of supplemental training programs, both alone and in combination with other interventions and treatment protocols (eg, mental health and biopsychosocial interventions), to optimize the effects of supplemental training in dancers.

Methodological Rigor and Scoring

The methodological rigor of the studies was generally low to moderate with weak strength of recommendation. Only 4 studies were of moderate quality and no study had high methodological rigor on the mDB criteria. Most studies also did not include confidence intervals for statistically significant results. When considering LOE and strength of recommendations, the general quality and quantity of the included studies was low. Bahr and Holme[66] estimate that 50 injured participants (not total participants) are needed to detect a moderate to strong association between a risk factor and injury. Given the low sample sizes in this review, the authors therefore believe that it is premature to associate injury risk and supplemental training.

As mentioned earlier, the authors recommend multicenter and longitudinal examinations with control groups because, although single-site studies may be more sensitive to site-specific effects,[67,68] multisite studies are more likely to include enough participants to allow researchers to examine the effects of multiple factors on performance and injury. However, these findings do not in themselves indicate any specific weakness in dance medicine and science, which are nascent.[17,18,69] The authors believe that these findings highlight the challenges of conducting research of high rigor in a niche field such as dance medicine and science, and advocate more work to help this underserved population. In support, Swain and colleagues[67] note that, because dancers are highly specialized, they are limited in numbers of potential participants. Thus, higher-quality, adequately powered studies and randomized controlled trials are needed to determine which interventions have the greatest effects on dancers' performance and injury risk.

Limitations

To the best of our knowledge, this is among the first reviews to examine supplemental training in dance across all levels of dance participation and genres using a systematic and rigorous approach. Despite using a comprehensive search strategy, the authors recognize that we may have missed relevant studies to include in this review. When developing the inclusion criteria, we decided to only include studies that incorporated current dancers, and did not use other populations that performed dance (eg, community dance exercise programs), possibly reducing the reach of the search. We also recognize that the small number of included studies and the overall low study quality could lead to bias in the conclusions.

Clinical Relevance

The clinical relevance of this study is that supplemental training programs that include multiple exercises and that are around 1 hour per session, implemented 2 to 3 times a week for 8 weeks, can enhance performance in dancers. Limited evidence exists for using supplemental training to reduce dancers' low back pain and injury risk. However, additional work is needed to confirm these observations in larger and longitudinal studies.

SUMMARY

Most studies included in this systematic review had small sample sizes and examined mostly collegiate women. Supplemental program type and dosage varied widely. Supplemental training effects were examined using discrete tests or fitness assessments not related specifically to dance, with only a few dance performance–specific measures. The studies had low to moderate methodological rigor with weak strength of recommendation. Supplemental training does seem to improve performance, with some evidence supporting decrease in low back injury and pain. Taken as a whole, review findings emphasize the complexity of implementing supplemental training in the niche dance population. Overall, practitioners can use review findings to advocate supplemental training inclusion in dancers' practice regimens to provide performance enhancement and injury risk reduction.

REFERENCES

1. Ambegaonkar JP, Schock CS, Caswell SV, et al. Lower extremity horizontal work but not vertical power predicts lower extremity injury in female collegiate dancers. J Strength Cond Res 2018;32(7):2018–24.
2. Koutedakis Y, Jamurtas T. The dancer as a performing athlete: physiological considerations. Sports Med 2004;34:651–61.
3. Angioi M, Metsios GS, Metsios G, et al. Fitness in contemporary dance: a systematic review. Int J Sports Med 2009;30(7):475–84.
4. Angioi M, Metsios G, Twitchett EA, et al. Effects of supplemental training on fitness and aesthetic competence parameters in contemporary dance: a randomised controlled trial. Med Probl Perform Art 2012;27(1):3–8.
5. Armstrong R, Relph N. Screening tools as a predictor of injury in dance: systematic literature review and meta-analysis. Sports Med Open 2018;4(1):33.
6. Kovácsné Bobály V, Szilágyi B, Kiss G, et al. Application and examination of the efficiency of a core stability training program among dancers. Eur J Integr Med 2016;8:3–7.
7. Brown A, Wells T, Schade ML, et al. Effects of plyometric training versus traditional weight training on strength, power, and aesthetic jumping ability in female collegiate dancers. J Dance Med Sci 2007;11(2):38–44.
8. Allen N, Nevill A, Brooks J, et al. Ballet injuries: injury incidence and severity over 1 year. J Orthop Sports Phys Ther 2012;42(9):781–90.
9. Bronner S, Ojofeitimi S, Rose D. Injuries in a modern dance company: Effect of comprehensive management on injury incidence and time loss. Am J Sports Med 2003;31(3):365–73.

10. Hincapié CA, Morton EJ, Cassidy JD. Musculoskeletal Injuries and Pain in Dancers: A Systematic Review. Arch Phys Med Rehabil 2008;89(9):1819–29.e6.
11. Trentacosta N, Sugimoto D, Micheli LJ. Hip and groin injuries in dancers: A systematic review. Sports Health 2017;9(5):422–7.
12. Bowling A. Injuries to dancers: prevalence, treatment, and perceptions of causes. BMJ 1989;298:731–4.
13. Luke AC, Kinney SA, D'Hemecourt PA, et al. Determinants of injury in young dancers. Med Probl Perform Art 2002;17(3):105–12.
14. Thomas H, Tarr J. Dancers' perceptions of pain and injury: positive and negative effects. J Dance Med Sci 2009;13(2):51–9.
15. Kerr ZY, Baugh CM, Hibberd EE, et al. Epidemiology of National Collegiate Athletic Association men's and women's swimming and diving injuries from 2009/2010 to 2013/2014. Br J Sports Med 2015;49(7):465–71.
16. Bradshaw EJ, Hume PA. Biomechanical approaches to identify and quantify injury mechanisms and risk factors in women's artistic gymnastics. Sports Biomech 2012;11(3):324–41.
17. Solomon RL, Micheli LJ. Technique as a consideration in modern dance injuries. Phys Sportsmed 1986;14(8):83–90.
18. Ambegaonkar JP. Dance medicine: at the university level. Dance Res J 2005; 37(2):113–9.
19. Wilson JC, Quinn BJ, Stratton CW, et al. Athletes doing arabesques: important considerations in the care of young dancers. Curr Sports Med Rep 2015;14(6): 448–54.
20. Liederbach M. Screening for functional capacity in dancers designing standardized, dance-specific injury prevention screening tools. J Dance Med Sci 1997; 1(3):93–106.
21. Koutedakis Y, Pacy PJ, Carson RJ. Health and fitness in professional dancers. Med Probl Perform Art 1997;12(1):23–7.
22. Wyon M. Preparing to perform: periodization and dance. J Dance Med Sci 2010; 14(2):67–72.
23. McCabe TR, Wyon MA, Ambegaonkar JP, et al. A bibliographic review of medicine and science research in DanceSport. Medical Problems of Performing Artists. 28(2) 70-79. Med Probl Perform Art 2013;28(2):79.
24. Twitchett EA, Angioi M, Koutedakis Y, et al. Do increases in selected fitness parameters affect the aesthetic aspects of classical ballet performance? Med Probl Perform Art 2011;26(1):35–8.
25. Allen N, Ribbans W, Nevill AM, et al. Musculoskeletal injuries in dance: a systematic review. Int J Phys Med Rehabil 2014;3(1):252.
26. Angioi M, Metsios GS, Twitchett E, et al. Association between selected physical fitness parameters and esthetic competence in contemporary dancers. J Dance Med Sci 2009;13(4):115–23.
27. Khan K, Brown J, Way S, et al. Overuse injuries in classical ballet. Sports Med 1995;19(5):341–57.
28. Koutedakis Y, Sharp NCC. Thigh-muscles strength training, dance exercise, dynamometry, and anthropometry in professional ballerinas. J Strength Cond Res 2004;18(4):714–8.
29. Stalder MA, Noble BJ, Wilkinson JG. The effects of supplemental weight training for ballet dancers. J Appl Sport Sci Res 1990;4(3):95–102.
30. Dowse RA, McGuigan MR, Harrison C. Effects of a resistance training intervention on strength, power, and performance in adolescent dancers. J Strength Cond Res 2017. https://doi.org/10.1519/JSC.0000000000002288.

31. Allen N, Wyon MA. Dance Medicine: Artist or athlete? SportEX Med 2008;35:6–9.
32. Liberati A, Altman DG, Tetzlaff J, et al. The PRISMA statement for reporting systematic reviews and meta-analyses of studies that evaluate health care interventions: explanation and elaboration. PLoS Med 2009;6(7):1–28.
33. Downs SH, Black N. The feasibility of creating a checklist for the assessment of the methodological quality both of randomised and non-randomised studies of health care interventions. J Epidemiol Community Health 1998;52(6):377–84.
34. Ebell MH, Siwek J, Weiss BD, et al. Strength of Recommendation Taxonomy (SORT): a patient-centered approach to grading evidence in the medical literature. J Am Board Fam Med 2004;17(1):59–67.
35. Oxford Centre of Evidence-Based Medicine. CEBM levels of evidence 2.1. Available at: http://www.cebm.net/wp-content/uploads/2014/06/CEBM-Levels-of-Evidence-2.1.pdf. Accessed December 14, 2017.
36. Roussel NA, Vissers D, Kuppens K, et al. Effect of a physical conditioning versus health promotion intervention in dancers: a randomized controlled trial. Man Ther 2014;19(6):562–8.
37. Karim A, Roddey T, Mitchell K, et al. Immediate effect of whole body vibration on sauté height and balance in female professional contemporary dancers a randomized controlled trial. J Dance Med Sci 2019;23(1):3–10.
38. Grossman G, Wilmerding MV. The Effect of Conditioning on the Height of Dancer's Extension in à la Seconde. J Dance Med Sci 2000;4(4):117–21.
39. Koutedakis Y, Hukam H, Metsios G, et al. The effects of three months of aerobic and strength training on selected performance- and fitness-related parameters in modern dance students. J Strength Cond Res 2007;21(3):808–12.
40. Stosic D, Slavoljub U, Pantelić S, et al. Effects of an exercise program on the coordination and explosive power of university dance students. Phys Educ Sport 2019;17(3):579–89.
41. Kalaycioglu T, Apostolopoulos NC, Goldere S, et al. Effect of a core stabilization training program on performance of ballet and modern dancers. J Strength Cond Res 2020;34(4):1166–75.
42. Pata D, Welsh T, Bailey J, et al. Improving turnout in university dancers. J Dance Med Sci 2014;18(4):169–77.
43. Watson T, Graning J, McPherson S, et al. Dance, balance and core muscle performance measures are improved following a 9-week core stabilization training program among competitive collegiate dancers. Int J Sports Phys Ther 2017;12(1):25–41.
44. Agel J, Klossner D. Epidemiologic review of collegiate acl injury rates across 14 sports: national collegiate athletic association injury surveillance system data 2004-05 through 2011-12. Br J Sports Med 2014;48(7):560.
45. Agel J, Arendt EA, Bershadsky B. Anterior cruciate ligament injury in national collegiate athletic association basketball and soccer a 13-year review. Am J Sports Med 2005;33(4):524–31.
46. Andreoli CV, Chiaramonti BC, Biruel E, et al. Epidemiology of sports injuries in basketball: integrative systematic review. BMJ Open Sport Exerc Med 2018;4(1):e000468.
47. Bennell K, Khan KM, Matthews B, et al. Hip and ankle range of motion and hip muscle strength in young female ballet dancers and controls. Br J Sports Med 1999;33(5):340–6.
48. Harley Y, Gibson A, Harley E, et al. Quadriceps strength and jumping efficiency in dancers. J Dance Med Sci 2002;6(3):87–94.

49. Ambegaonkar JP, Caswell SV, Winchester JB, et al. Upper-body muscular endurance in female university-level modern dancers: a pilot study. J Dance Med Sci 2012;16(1):3–7.
50. Jacobs CL, Hincapié CA, Cassidy JD. Musculoskeletal injuries and pain in dancers: a systematic review update. J Dance Med Sci 2012;16(2):74–84.
51. Bronner S, Worthen L. The demographics of dance in the united states. J Dance Med Sci 1999;3(4):151–3.
52. Bronner S, Wood L. Impact of touring, performance schedule, and definitions on 1-year injury rates in a modern dance company. J Sports Sci 2017;35(21):2093–104.
53. Orishimo KF, Kremenic IJ, Pappas E, et al. Comparison of landing biomechanics between male and female professional dancers. Am J Sports Med 2009;37(11):2187–93.
54. Cahalan R, O'Sullivan K. Job satisfaction of professional Irish dancers. J Dance Med Sci 2013;17(4):139–49.
55. Sheth S, Fauntroy V, Ambegaonkar JP. Physical activity in Kathak using biosensors: A pilot study. Loud Applause 2020;3(2):4–9.
56. Ojofeitimi S, Bronner S, Woo H. Injury incidence in hip hop dance. Scand J Med Sci Sports 2012;22(3):347–55.
57. Cho CH, Song KS, Min BW, et al. Musculoskeletal injuries in break-dancers. Injury 2009;40(11):1207–11.
58. Cahalan R, Bargary N, O'Sullivan K. Pain and Injury in Elite Adolescent Irish Dancers A Cross-Sectional Study. J Dance Med Sci 2018;22(2):91–9.
59. Liiv H, Wyon MA, Jürimäe T, et al. Anthropometry, somatotypes, and aerobic power in ballet, contemporary dance, and dancesport. Med Probl Perform Art 2013;28(4):207–11.
60. Clarke F, Koutedakis Y, Wilson M, et al. Balance in Theatrical Dance Performance: A Systematic Review. Med Probl Perform Art 2018;33(4):275–85.
61. Oxfeldt M, Overgaard K, Hvid LG, et al. Effects of plyometric training on jumping, sprint performance, and lower body muscle strength in healthy adults: A systematic review and meta-analyses. Scand J Med Sci Sports 2019;29(10):1453–65.
62. Slimani M, Chamari K, Miarka B, et al. Effects of plyometric training on physical fitness in team sport athletes: a systematic review. J Hum Kinet 2016;53:231–47.
63. Ambegaonkar JP, Caswell SV, Winchester JB, et al. Balance comparisons between female dancers and active nondancers. Res Q Exerc Sport 2013;84(1):24–9.
64. Twitchett E, Brodrick A, Nevill AM, et al. Does physical fitness affect injury occurrence and time loss due to injury in elite vocational ballet students? J Dance Med Sci 2010;14(1):26–31.
65. Fauntroy V, Nolton E, Ambegaonkar JP. Health-related quality of life (HRQoL) measures used in dance: a systematic review. Int J Sports Phys Ther 2020;15(3):1–10.
66. Bahr R, Holme I. Risk factors for sports injuries–a methodological approach. Br J Sports Med 2003;37(5):384–92.
67. Swain CTV, Bradshaw EJ, Ekegren CL, et al. The epidemiology of low back pain and injury in dance: a systematic review. J Orthop Sports Phys Ther 2019;49(4):239–52.
68. Kahn MG, Raebel MA, Glanz JM, et al. A pragmatic framework for single-site and multisite data quality assessment in electronic health record-based clinical research. Med Care 2012;50(Suppl):S21–9.
69. Schon LC, Weinfeld SB. Lower extremity musculoskeletal problems in dancers. Curr Opin Rheumatol 1996;8(2):130–42.

On-site Clinical Care for Professional Dance Companies

Kathleen Bower, PT, DPT[a],*, Carina M. Nasrallah, MS, ATC[b],
Bené Barrera, BS, ATC[c], Kevin E. Varner, MD[d], Alex Y. Han, MD[d]

KEYWORDS

- Dance • Performing arts medicine • Multidisciplinary • Health care • Injuries
- Injury prevention • Wellness • Health

KEY POINTS

- Best practice for care of professional dancers involves an interdisciplinary approach with streamlined referrals and communication between a network of health care providers familiar with the unique demands of the professional dance setting.
- Incorporating movement specialists into the dancer wellness team promotes dancer health and fitness, as well as reducing injury when cross-training principles are properly implemented.
- On-site health care is cost-effective for dance companies by reducing injury rates and mitigating workers' compensation premiums.
- Designing a highly effective dance medicine program involves nurturing a culture in which the dancers, health care team, and artistic staff/administration are actively engaged in promoting injury prevention and supporting injured dancers' journeys to recovery.

INTRODUCTION

Over the last 30 years, most major dance companies have developed extensive on-site dance medicine clinics staffed with health care and wellness teams to handle the growing load of musculoskeletal (MSK) complaints, whereas smaller companies have also worked to provide their dancers with direct access to health care.[1,2] On-site care provided by physicians, physical therapists, athletic trainers, and massage therapists allows the effective management of MSK complaints, whereas regular visits from a company physician can provide dancers with their initial consults into the

[a] Miami City Ballet, 2200 Liberty Avenue, Miami Beach, FL 33139, USA; [b] Houston Methodist Orthopedics & Sports Medicine, 601 Preston Street, Houston, TX 77002, USA; [c] Houston Methodist Orthopedics & Sports Medicine, 18400 Katy Fwy – Suite 200, Houston, TX 77094, USA; [d] Houston Methodist Orthopedics & Sports Medicine, 6445 Main Street, Suite 2500, Houston, TX 77030, USA
* Corresponding author.
E-mail address: KBowerDPT@gmail.com

Phys Med Rehabil Clin N Am 32 (2021) 137–153
https://doi.org/10.1016/j.pmr.2020.09.002
1047-9651/21/© 2020 Elsevier Inc. All rights reserved.

broader health care system. As with other professional and collegiate teams, there are many benefits in having a multidisciplinary approach to care for professional dance companies.[3] This approach provides unparalleled health care to dancers for injury prevention and treatment, for both elite performance and long-term health, as well as financial benefits to the company by decreasing injury incidence, lost days, and workers' compensation claims.[4–7]

The goal of a multidisciplinary health care team (HCT) is to optimize the health and well-being of the dancers through comprehensive health management while simultaneously enhancing their performance. Management of a dancer's care encompasses MSK evaluation, triage, physician appointments, imaging, rehabilitation, and alternative therapies. This dynamic collaboration allows a close relationship with the dancer, physician, and on-site HCT. Companies have also shifted into providing preventive care through screening, wellness interventions, and conditioning classes, leading to an overall reduction in time-loss injures.[5,8,9]

This article discusses the development of an on-site clinic to meet the needs of a company, selection of appropriate equipment and modalities, overview of health care and wellness services, and effective communication between the HCT and the company staff.

FACILITY AND PROGRAM DEVELOPMENT

The development or renovation of an on-site health care facility for a professional dance company is affected by multiple factors:

- Company's goals and needs
- Company's budget
- Number of dancers
- Size of space (square meters)
- Location of facility
- Staffing requirements
- Special design elements (ceiling height, door placement, footprint of space)

At minimum, the planning process should include the facilities manager, the primary on-site clinician, and the general manager. For new builds, a planning committee and executive administrators may also be involved.

The implementation of the on-site health care program should have a clear purpose to ensure the facility is designed to fulfill the needs as identified by the dance company. Having assessed the factors listed earlier, the organization can then determine their primary goals and functions for the program, such as:

- Mitigation of workers' compensation claims and/or premiums
- Reduction of time-loss injuries
- Injury prevention and management
- Long-term health and wellness
- Performance readiness and optimization
- Expedited care and referrals

Once the goals of the on-site health care program have been established, the next step is to identify the services to be provided:

- Triage of injury/illness
- Treatment of MSK injury
- Preseason screenings
- Wellness consultations

- Strength and conditioning programs
- Education workshops/seminars

The facility's layout, capacity, and design should contribute to optimal safety, function, and ergonomics for the on-site clinicians and dancers. When designing an on-site clinic, it is essential that the facility meet local building and safety ordinances but also provides the components of a high-performance health care facility. The facility should be designated into dry and wet areas.[10] **Table 1** provides an example of a layout of an on-site health care facility.

Dry areas include:

- General treatment and evaluation area
- Private examination area
- Rehabilitation/therapeutic area
- Taping and bandaging area
- Program administration/office area
- Storage area

Wet areas include:

- Hydrocollator
- Freezer
- Washer/dryer
- Whirlpool and hydrotherapies

For safety, all areas within the on-site facility should be provided with:

- Adequate lighting

Table 1
Design functions required for dry and wet areas

General treatment and evaluation area	Semiprivate area designated for assessment, modality application, treatments, and so forth
Examination area	Private area designated for examinations, massage, consultations, and so forth
Rehabilitation/therapeutic area	Open area for therapeutic exercise and equipment. Composite flooring or mats for plyometric activity, weights, or floor protection of equipment. May also house auxiliary equipment, including weights, cardio equipment, Gyrotonic and Pilates equipment
Taping and bandaging area	Open area that may be kept separate for improved traffic flow; may also be wound care and self-care area. This area may also double for supply storage
Traffic areas	Pathways designated by cleared floor space or half walls
Program administration/ office area	Size dependent on number of staff. Should be open or have windows for complete line of sight of entire facility. Secure area for storing of sensitive items, electronics, and documentation
Storage area	Adequate space for storing supplies and equipment. Should include cleared floor space with use of cabinets, hooks, and so forth
Hydrotherapy area	Enclosed space because of noise but visible line of sight via half walls and windows. Additional drainage, larger water fill pipes and drains, raised electric outlets, ground fault inhibitors, nonslip flooring, water mixers if using whirlpools, and seating required

- Line of sight for clinician supervision
- Wheelchair-accessible doors
- Handwashing/sanitizing stations
- Sufficient and properly placed power supply sources with grounded fault circuit interrupter

Specific needs by area include:

- Sharps container and biohazard disposal within general treatment and taping
- Nonslip flooring for wet areas
- Composite flooring for rehabilitation and conditioning areas
- Adequate ceiling height for rehabilitation and conditioning areas
- Specified ventilation needs to address humidity of wet area
- Independent lock security of general evaluation/treatment area and clinical administration/office area

The facility should allow for open accessibility to all dancers through a main door and potentially other dancer-only areas, such as dressing rooms or studios. Traffic flow within the facility should be adequate for dancers to move around safely, avoiding possible injury of moving bodies, equipment, projectiles, and/or tripping hazards. Lips of flooring should be addressed with sloping attachment pieces or definitively marked. Security of the facility should be independent of that of the building as well as any administrative, electronics, modalities or Health Insurance Portability and Accountability Act (HIPAA) sensitive materials.[10]

All aforementioned components are integral to the overall layout, design, and flow of the facility. These components should be assessed regardless of new-build or existing structure when implementing a safe, effective, and high-performance health care facility on site (**Fig. 1**).

BUDGETING AND STRATEGIC PLANNING

The resources and services provided through an on-site health care program must revolve around sound budgeting practices and strategic planning, ensuring continued

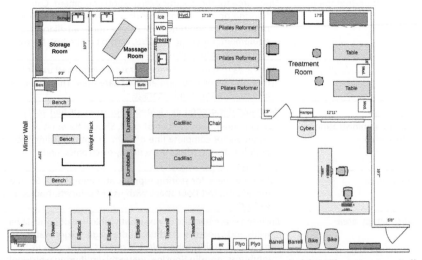

Fig. 1. On-site health care facility by Houston Methodist Hospital (HMH) at Houston Ballet.

growth and viability. Each company's budget should be tailored to its needs and is typically under the management of the head clinician and/or the company general manager. A facility manager may also be involved with management of capital expenses and facility maintenance, such as remodels, housekeeping services, large equipment purchases, and equipment maintenance.

Operational Budgeting

Dance companies need to determine their budgets based on providing in-house clinicians or contracted services from an outside source, such as a hospital, physical therapy clinic, or independent clinician. Defining the program's primary goals, staffing needs, and overall budget helps determine whether services are provided in house or through contracted partners.

Depending on a company's financial structure and the size of the program, the budget system may use program, line item, fixed, or variable budgeting.[10] In some cases, a combination of budget styles may be implemented, an example being a zero-based budget with a maximum cap or fixed budget for the fiscal or calendar year. Determining whether the program's budget is to rely on quarterly cash availability or an agreed-on fixed cap for the year further aids in deciphering the type of budget system best suited.

Types of Expenses

Once the budget style is determined, the head clinician can make clear justifications for allocation of resources based on expense types: operational budget and equipment/supplies and services budget (**Fig. 2**). Both budgets involve short-term expenses on a quarterly or annual basis. The operational budget pertains to daily operations involving salaries, benefits, administrative costs, and office operations.[11] It is also encouraged that employers contribute to or reimburse clinicians through the operations budget for professional development and continuing education that directly supports the program. The equipment/supplies and services budget pertains to expendable and nonexpendable supplies, equipment, and services. Annual equipment maintenance, repairs, and modality calibrations should be included when planning this budget.

EQUIPMENT AND MODALITIES

The facility should be equipped to include various modalities, training equipment, and tools for the dancers to use for their individual goals and treatment plans. Equipment and modalities provided within the on-site facility should be chosen according to the program's needs, the clinician's scope of practice, and the budget outlined for the program.

Whether designating new build or retrofitting an on-site health care space, ensuring adequate floor area (square meters), ceiling height, and power sources for equipment should not be overlooked. Because it is common for many companies' on-site facilities to be shared between multiple disciplines, it is important to determine equipment based on practitioners' needs. Large equipment may include, but is not limited to, cardio machines, weight racks, Pilates trapeze table, reformers, Gyrotonics towers, and jump-and-stretch board (**Table 2**). Accurate measurements prove both time and cost-effective when planning, purchasing, and installing equipment.

Modality selections should be determined by the scope of practice and the skillset of the clinicians as well as dancer use. Examples of modalities commonly used in on-site clinics include, but are not limited to, electric stimulation, ultrasonography,

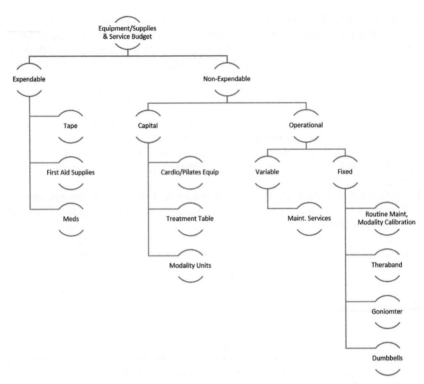

Fig. 2. Equipment and services budgeting. Equip., equipment; Maint., maintenance.

infrared laser, massage, instrument-assisted soft tissue manipulation, manual therapy, thermotherapy/cryotherapy, and dry needling.

SERVICES

The on-site HCT for a professional dance company is responsible for providing and coordinating a variety of services, including preventive care, assessment and referral, injury care, as well as rehabilitation and return to dance (**Fig. 3**).

Preventive Care

Offering preventive care can promote a well-rounded experience that can be tailored to the dancers and their specific needs, with an emphasis on long-term health and career longevity. Preventive care can include, but is not limited to, preseason physicals or screenings, daily or weekly access to on-site practitioners, and educational programs.

Preseason physicals or preparticipation examinations (PPEs) have been used in sports medicine for decades and are becoming more widely integrated into dance medicine practices, especially among professional dance companies. The goal of the PPE is to determine the dancer's current health status and identify any potential risk factors that may affect the dancer's ability to safely engage in the physical demands of the profession.[12–14] Additional advantages to the PPE include:

- Entry into the health care system for new dancers
- Development of rapport between health care provider and dancer

Table 2 Equipment and modalities	
General treatment and evaluation area	Treatment tables, cabinetry, modality carts, various modalities (electric stimulation, Game Ready, ultrasonography, pneumatic devices, infrared laser, dry needling, IASTM, and so forth), diagnostic tools, educational tools/models, bolsters, sharps container, biohazard disposal, and so forth
Examination area	Examination table, sink, work area, cabinetry, other examination equipment, consultation equipment, educational models, and so forth
Rehabilitation/therapeutic area	Cardio, strength and conditioning, Pilates, Gyrotonics equipment, mats, foam rollers, weight rack, bands, kettlebells, mirror, plyometric boxes, and so forth
Taping and bandaging area	Taping table, biohazard disposal, taping supplies, wound care supplies, sink, cabinetry
Traffic areas	Cleared areas for traffic flow that are not easily congested. Having a check-in kiosk for treatment could be located at the entryway
Program administration/ office area	Office or designated workstation for administrative work, documentation, and program development with computers, printers, secure storage, secure Internet/software access, phone, and so forth
Storage area	Cabinetry/shelving and hanging space for back stock supplies and equipment
Hydrotherapy area	Whirlpool, fridge/freezer, washing/drying unit, ice machine, hydrocollator, and so forth

Abbreviation: IASTM, instrument-assisted soft tissue mobilization.

- Identification of individual factors that might contribute to injury risk
- Dancer education on individual wellness and injury prevention strategies

Despite increased implementation of the PPE among professional companies, several barriers are often cited, including time and money constraints, difficulty gaining support from the dancers and staff, and lack of research.[12,15] Partnering with a hospital system and health care entity or community provider off site may provide access to additional resources for a PPE event compared with an on-site event.

Management of MSK complaints constitutes most on-site care. Advocating for early reporting and detection with an on-site health care program may reduce the number of injuries causing modifications and time loss.[16–18] A multidisciplinary approach to managing MSK complains may include therapeutic interventions, chiropractic care, strength and conditioning, nutrition services, and mental health consultations. Implementing an individualized, multifaceted management plan combined with early reporting may effectively show a reduction of injury rates and improved health practices.[19]

Dancer education programs offer a cost-efficient and time-efficient mode of preventive care. An on-site program can include educational forums, written resources, or interactive sessions on a wide variety of wellness topics as well as dancer requests. Implementation of educational opportunities can encourage diverse insight, expand knowledge of resources, and promote buy-in from the company dancers.[20,21] Furthermore, such programs organized by the HCT better ensure that the dancers have access to reliable, quality information and recommendations for best practice.

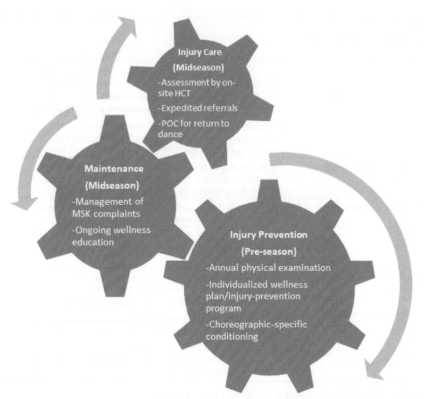

Fig. 3. The function of an on-site dancer wellness program. POC, plan of care.

Assessment and Referral

The HCT should strive to cultivate an environment where dancers access available wellness resources often and have clear understanding of their role in preventing and managing their injuries. The on-site HCT is the liaison between the dancer, the supervising physicians, and any additional allied health care professionals or outside resources. Continuity of care is a primary advantage provided by on-site programs. The rapport between the on-site HCT and dancer can help to:

- Reduce the stress of seeking a reputable provider
- Expedite care and accessibility
- Provide a broader scope of resources
- Allow for specialized care when needed

Injury Care

Injury care rendered by the on-site practitioner involves a multistep process. Establishing an injury care policy is essential to overall compliance and consistency of quality. The professional dance setting is a competitive, high-stress, and fluid environment. Such characteristics, when not regulated by an injury protocol, may result in confusion, frustration, and inefficiency of care.

Acute injury care requires a properly qualified clinician to perform a thorough assessment of the injury and mechanism while bearing in mind the dancer's individual medical history. On completion of the assessment, the clinician can determine the appropriate plan of care. The step-by-step process of pain management, referral, plan development, and communication of limitations or removal from participation is essential to a positive outcome. The acute injury can be traumatic and even devastating, especially if it involves time loss or surgical intervention.[22] A clear plan of action created by the on-site clinician, dancer, and staff is crucial in providing high-quality care. An injury plan may include the following:

1. Injury assessment and determination of severity
2. Management of symptoms; referral if needed
3. Communication with staff regarding severity of injury and limitations only
   a. Generate worker's compensation injury claim (if needed)
4. Development of plan of care
5. Progression through plan of care; ongoing communication about dancer limitations and expected return to dance
   a. Formal meetings pertaining to injury/plan/progression/limitations between dancer and staff may also include clinician for consistency and clarity
6. Initiation of injury-specific return-to-dance protocol
7. Clear and concise communication between dancer, clinicians, and staff for clearance to return to dance

Subacute, chronic, and overuse injury care can require prolonged maintenance measures because of the complex nature of these injuries. They require a high level of compliance, consistency, and self-sufficiency from the dancer. A dancer may need to maintain a modified volume or intensity for longer while striving to balance the current workload and recovery. Addressing these injuries requires realistic goal setting and frequent reassessment of the dancer's progress. Communication and understanding between clinicians, dancer, and staff is vital to the recovery of chronic and overuse injuries.

PERFORMANCE AND EVENT COVERAGE
The Backstage Clinic

Before preparing a backstage treatment area, it is recommended to coordinate with the company production management team to determine the size, location, and any additional medical supplies that may be available at the venue. In some situations, there may be specific space or travel limitations that affect what type of medical supplies can be transported or stored backstage (eg, flying with supplies vs shipping). Considerations to review with the production or company managers before backstage setup include:

- Dancer-patient privacy
- Size of treatment area/clinic
- Proximity of treatment area to stage and/or dancer warm-up area
- Availability of ice and other medical equipment (eg, automated external defibrillators, wheelchairs, spine boards, oxygen)
- Additional emergency or medical personnel that might cover events at the venue

The Backstage Medical Kit

When providing performance coverage, clinicians may not have direct access to a fully stocked clinic or medical supplies. Therefore, a transportable medical bag or kit may need to be prepared.[23,24] In addition to first-aid supplies and basic examination equipment, clinicians may also want to have some preferred modalities or manual therapy tools available. For longer tours or residencies, it might be advised to bring additional rehabilitation supplies for dancers needing therapeutic exercise programs. **Table 3** includes a list of supplies for a well-prepared medical kit that can be adjusted to meet the clinicians' specific needs.

In addition, a physician may consider bringing the following:

- Syringes/needles
- Scalpel
- Suture kit
- Prescription medications
- Prescription pad

The Medical Emergency Action Plan

Catastrophic injuries and life-threatening medical emergencies are not common in the dance studio or theater, but it is critical to remember that dancers are elite athletes and

Table 3
Equipment for backstage and tours

Evaluation	General first aid
• Paper and pen	• Alcohol swabs and povidone iodine swabs
• Treatment/evaluation table	• Bandage scissors
• Pin light or flashlight	• Bandages, sterile/nonsterile, Band-Aids
• Pin or other sharp object for sensory testing	• Disinfectant
• Reflex hammer	• Gloves
• Sideline concussion evaluation tool	• Sharps box and biohazard bag
• Oto-ophthalmoscope	• Steri-Strips/skin glue
• Oral/rectal thermometer	• Wound wash materials (eg, sterile normal saline)
• Tongue depressors	• Eye kit (eg, eyewash, contact case and solution, mirror)
• Weight scale	• Blister care materials
• Glucose monitor	• Nail clippers
	• Skin lubricant
	• Skin glue
Cardiopulmonary	Medications (OTC)
• Stethoscope	• Topical antibiotic
• Blood pressure cuff	• Local anesthetic
• Epinephrine	• NSAIDs
• Mouth-to-mouth mask	• Antacid
• Short-acting beta-agonist inhaler	• Antidiarrheal
• Automated external defibrillator	• Antihistamine
	• Sleep aid
Modalities	Bracing and splinting
• Skin emollient	• Extremity splints
• Dry needling/ acupuncture supplies	• Sling
• Cupping kit	• Crutches
• TENS unit	• Walking boot
• Cold packs or ice cooler	• Semirigid cervical collar
• Traction strap	• Taping supplies
• IASTM tools	
• Resistance bands	
• Trigger point balls and foam rollers	

Abbreviations: NSAIDs, nonsteroidal antiinflammatory drugs; OTC, over the counter; TENS, transcutaneous electrical nerve stimulation.

not immune to catastrophic injury. One of the most important written procedures for on-site providers is an emergency action plan (EAP) that outlines how medical emergencies will be managed within a dance institution or performance venue. The plan should be clear, comprehensive, and adaptable to a variety of scenarios.[25,26]

In the case of an emergency, roles need to be delegated and the parties should know their responsibilities in advance. Instructors, staff, administrators, any on-site or off-site medical personnel (ie, athletic trainers, physical therapists, physicians), and the local emergency medical services (EMS) team should be familiar with the venue-specific EAP. The EAP should answer the following:

- Who will call EMS?
- Who will perform the initial evaluation?
- Where is emergency equipment located (automated external defibrillators, oxygen, splints, and so forth)
- Who will fetch emergency equipment?
- Who will escort EMS into the facility?
- Who determines whether the show needs to be stopped or casting changed midperformance?

An EAP should be reviewed and revised as needed at least once a year with staff and medical personnel. A well-designed and rehearsed EAP reduces time-costly errors and ensures that communication and order are maintained in an emergency situation.

THE DANCE MEDICINE HEALTH CARE TEAM

Objectives of the dance medicine team:

- Coordinate preparticipation screening and evaluation to determine dancers' readiness for work demands.
- Evaluate and manage acute and nonacute injuries that occur during classes, rehearsals, and performances.
- Communicate with the dancers and artistic staff about safe parameters for participation following injury or illness.
- Rehabilitate and recondition dancers following injury for a safe return to dance.
- Provide education and evidence-based resources that are relevant to professional dancers.
- Recognize mental health and nutritional crises and intervene appropriately.
- Coordinate referrals and facilitate communication among other members of the allied HCT.
- Maintain proper documentation and administrative tasks.

The Multidisciplinary Approach to Dancer-Centered Care

The multidisciplinary HCT approach for providing care to athletic organizations has been well described.[3,26,27] From the collegiate to the professional level, a myriad of sports have used this approach, but historically there has been a limited team approach for health care in dance medicine. As with traditional professional sports, there is a significant need to reduce or prevent injuries, diminish the impact on the dancers, and mitigate the significant costs associated with those injuries. Sporer and Windt[28] noted that, "It is not enough simply to have a group of individual practitioners surrounding the athlete and calling it an integrated performance team. Integration is an active process that requires commitment, time, teamwork and leadership."[28] Critically, this is dancer-centered care and not only involves the multidisciplinary HCT but places the dancers at the center of a shared decision-making process.

With expansion in medical knowledge and increasing subspecialization in medicine, comprehensive care for elite dancers requires diverse multidisciplinary teams. These teams include orthopedic surgeons, physiatrists, primary care sports medicine physicians, athletic trainers, physical therapists, chiropractors, massage therapists, acupuncturists, nutritionists, and sports psychologists. Typically, there is a lead or head team physician, which is often an orthopedic surgeon, physiatrist, or primary care sports medicine physician with a knowledge of dance medicine. In particular, the head physician should have the expertise to appropriately guide return-to-dance decisions and determine clearance for full duty.[29,30]

Team Approach to Dancer Wellness

Most on-site facilities not only house members of the HCT but also house members of a wellness team (WT). The WT may include a Pilates instructor, Gyrotonics instructor, therapeutic class instructor, strength and conditioning coach, massage therapist, and so forth. Such roles play an essential part in dancer care, injury rehabilitation, injury prevention, and performance enhancement, thus it is just as essential that the HCT and the WT work in tandem when coordinating dancer care (**Fig. 4**).[31]

Understanding the roles of each discipline and the appropriate allocation and referral of such resources can lead the dancers to a better experience and more

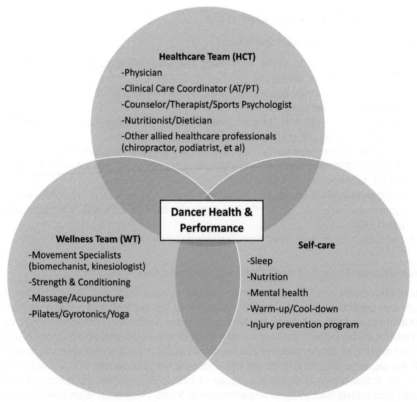

Fig. 4. The team approach to dancer wellness. AT, athletic trainer; PT, physical therapist.

positive outcomes as they progress through their injuries and their careers. The HCT and WT relationship should promote the communication of the goals set by the HCT for a particular dancer at a particular benchmark within the injury or health process. In reciprocity, the WT should be able to communicate any observations or concerns noted during the team's interactions with the dancer to the HCT.

Coverage Considerations

When determining the type and number of clinicians to staff the on-site facilities, consideration should be given to types and availability of the services to be offered, as well as the number of dancers accessing those services. Among professional and elite sports teams in North America, athletic trainers (athletic therapists) are typically the primary on-site clinicians managing the athletes' care. Outside of the United States and Canada, this role might be filled by a sports physical therapist (physiotherapist). Among North American professional ballet companies, both athletic trainers and physical therapists often serve in that capacity while working closely with a supervising or head team physician and other allied health care professionals.

The number of on-site clinical staff is determined by hours of on-site care for the dancers. Larger companies ($\geq$50 dancers) benefit from having a minimum of 40 h/wk of on-site coverage, but additional staffing could provide expanded treatment hours and services. Smaller companies (<30) who rehearse 6 h/d or less may warrant fewer hours per week or the equivalent of a part-time HCT. At present there are no guidelines outlining appropriate medical coverage for professional dance companies, but a well-developed program should have clinical staff on site anytime the dancers are participating in company activities (class, rehearsal, or performance) as well as any additional treatment times before or after those events. Coverage during layoffs, dark days, and holidays should be determined based on need and may vary depending on the size of the company and number of active injuries. Companies that tour nationally or internationally should consider bringing a company HCT member or making arrangements for a local athletic trainer or physical therapist to provide coverage for the dancers while on tour.

Any clinician working with a professional ballet company should be familiar with the dancers' vernacular and dance terminology, as well as having an understanding of the unique physical and mental demands of the art form as a profession. This familiarity is crucial to the dancer-patient's experience and perceptions of care.[32,33] All members of the HCT should participate in continuing education courses, fellowships, or residencies within dance medicine to be familiar with this subspecialty.

Establishing Additional Health Care Resources

Specialized physicians and allied health care specialties can be of great value to the on-site HCT, especially if they have a knowledge of or interest in dance medicine and show a willingness to work as part of the team. Incorporating specialists such obstetrics and gynecology, endocrinology, psychiatry, ophthalmology, and otolaryngology can provide great insight and increase medical accessibility for the dancers.

Developing a relationship within the local health care network can be a valuable component of the dancer's off-site health care access. This relationship is where a hospital system or health care entity can provide additional support that may otherwise not be available. Having an interested and engaged team of allied health care providers in the community can assist in expediting the speed and quality of care, including diagnostic imaging as well as additional treatment options for the dancers. These relationships also provide dancers with the latest technology and advancements in standard of care for screening, diagnosis, and treatments, which may not be available on site.

DANCER PRIVACY AND WORKERS' COMPENSATION
Health Insurance Portability and Accountability Act and Protected Health Information

Within the dance culture, many dancers still perceive a stigma regarding injury and the potential repercussions of seeking care, which may make them unwilling to tell their employers about injury occurrence or request modifications to their work load.[34] This stigma may lead to delayed reporting, increased injury severity, and time loss. Integrated support and communication between the HCT, dancer, and artistic staff can be an essential part of a dancers return.[28] It is necessary for the HCT to respect HIPAA practices and not disclose information without verbal or written consent from the dancer.

Because of the high demands of a professional dancer's schedule, the HCT has a responsibility to share essential information only as it pertains to the dancer's specific work limitations and expected return to full duty. The HCT can provide a notice of disclosure for each dancer that provides the understanding as to what information is discussed between the HCT and artistic staff. Notice of disclosures does not have to be signed for each injury but may be a general form provided for all injuries that are sustained during a season. The dancer has the right to revoke this blanket disclosure at any time. Best practices support a collaborative model where the dancer is an active participant in communications and decisions between the artistic staff and HCT. This collaboration facilitates compliance, effective communication, improved health care experiences, and better dancer outcomes.[28,31,32]

Workers' Compensation

One of the primary benefits of on-site care is to mitigate workers' compensation premiums through shared risk.[4] In professional dance companies in the United States, workers' compensation premiums are calculated by using the companies' previous 3 years of injury claims data to determine the experience modification ratio (EMR), the rate (average risk compared with other similar businesses), and the total payroll divided by 100: Premium = risk × (payroll/100) × EMR. The EMR assists insurance companies in understanding both past cost of injuries and probable risk of future injuries. The review for determination of the EMR includes the total amount paid out in claims and number of injuries reported, with more weight going to total number of injuries reported. If dance companies choose to assume some of the risk by providing on-site care for smaller, chronic injuries primarily treated with therapy, the larger, more serious or time-loss injuries are reported to workers' compensation, allowing a decrease in the total EMR.[1] Studies involving several major US dance companies have shown that providing on-site care decreases or maintains an EMR to less than 1.0 and leads to lower premiums and reduced medical expenses.[4,6]

Most injuries sustained by professional dancers are work related.[34-37] Although each state has its own laws governing workers' compensation, the general reporting guidelines and internal reporting procedures are similar. Workers' compensation requires specific information pertaining to the mechanism, date, location, and circumstances of the injury, including the suspected diagnosis. Most of this information can be provided by the on-site HCT or dancer and reported to workers' compensation through encrypted methods by the company manager or head clinician.

SUMMARY

On-site clinics can offer great financial benefit to dance companies as well a comfortable environment where the dancers can receive a high level of specialized care. A strong HCT and WT under the direction of a primary on-site clinician and physician can assist in expediting patient care, facilitate communication between the dancers and company staff, as well as return the dancers to full duty in a timely manner. Although an on-site facility and program as described earlier does have a financial impact on the company, it should provide an overall advantage by assuming some of the risk, mitigating worker's compensation premiums, and decreasing the amount of time lost to injury. This dynamic approach should deliver an improved health care experience and, ultimately, healthier dancers.

DISCLOSURE

The authors have nothing to disclose.

REFERENCES

1. Solomon R, Micheli L, Solomon J, et al. The "cost" of injuries in a professional ballet company: Anatomy of a season. Med Probl Perform Ar 1995;10(3):3–10.
2. Allen N, Nevill A, Brooks J, et al. Ballet injuries: injury incidence and severity over 1 year. J Orthop Sports Phys Ther 2012;42(9):781–90.
3. Buran MP, Alexander J, et al. An exploratory study in to the development of a multidisciplinary team in elite level cricket: a thematic analysis. J Research in Sports Med 2019;4(2):1–10.
4. Solomon R, Soloman J, Micheli LJ, et al. The "cost" of injuries in a professional ballet company: A five-year study. Med Probl Perform Ar 1999;14(4):164–70.
5. Allen N, Nevill AM, Brooks JH, et al. The effect of a comprehensive injury audit program on injury incidence in ballet: a 3-year prospective study. Clin J Sport Med 2013;23(5):373–8.
6. Bronner S, Ojofeitimi S. Injuries in a Modern Dance Company Effect of Comprehensive Management on Injury Incidence and Cost. J Dance Med Sci 2011;15(3):116–22.
7. Garrick JG, Requa RK. Ballet injuries. An analysis of epidemiology and financial outcome. Am J Sports Med 1993;21:586–90.
8. Russell JA. Preventing dance injuries: current perspectives. Open Access J Sports Med 2013;4:199–210.
9. Vera AM, Barrera BD. An injury prevention program for professional ballet: A randomized controlled investigation. Orthop J Sports Med 2020;8(7). 2325967120937643.
10. Konin J, Ray R. Management strategies in athletic training. 4th edition. Champaign (IL): Human Kinetic; 2011. p. 132–8, 157-179, 198-206.
11. Harrelson GL, Gardner G, Winterstein AP. Administrative topics in athletic training. Thorofare (NJ): SLACK Inc.; 2009. p. 45–50, 115-119.
12. Kilburn CM, Singh H, Makowski A, et al. Perspectives of Physical Therapists Regarding the Use and Value of Screening Assessments and Preventative Programs for Elite-Level Dancers. J Dance Med Sci 2020;24(1):3–11.
13. Novosel B, Sekulic D, Peric M, et al. Injury Occurrence and Return to Dance in Professional Ballet: Prospective Analysis of Specific Correlates. Int J Environ Res Public Health 2019;16(5):765.

14. Lee L, Reid D, Cadwell J, et al. Injury incidence, dance exposure and the use of the movement competency screen (MCS) to identify variable associated with injury in full-time pre-professional dancers. Int J Sports Phys Ther 2017;12(3): 352–70.

15. Armstrong R, Relph N. Screening tools as a predictor of injury in dance: Systematic literature review and meta-analysis. Sports Med Open 2018;4(1):33.

16. Bronner S, Ojofeitimi S, Mayers L. Comprehensive surveillance of dance injuries a proposal for uniform reporting guidelines for professional companies. J Dance Med Sci 2006;10(3&4):69–80.

17. Ambegaonkar JP, Caswell SV. Development and implementation of an in-house healthcare program for university-level performing artists. Work 2011;40(3): 261–8.

18. Allen N, Wj R, Nevill AM, et al. Musculoskeletal Injuries in Dance: A Systematic Review. Int J Phys Med Rehabil 2014;3(1):252.

19. Kinney S, McCrystal T, Owen M, et al. The effect of physical therapist involvement in the diagnosis and treatment of youth and adolescent dancers' injuries. J Dance Med Sci 2018;22(2):81–3.

20. Clark T, Gupta A, Ho CH. Developing a dancer wellness program employing developmental evaluation. Front Psychol 2014;5:731.

21. Cardinal MK. Wellness Education for Dancers. J Phys Educ Recreat Dance 2009; 80(5):29–39.

22. Adam MU, Brassington GS, Matheson GO. Psychological factors associated with performance-limiting injuries in professional ballet dancers. J Dance Med Sci 2004;8(2):43–6, 104.

23. Daniels JM, Kary J, Lane JA. Optimizing the sideline medical bag preparing for school and community sports events. Phys Sportsmed 2005;33(12):9–16.

24. Derman W. Guidelines for the composition of the travelling medical kit for sports medicine professionals. Int Sports Med J 2011;12(3):125–32.

25. Courson R. Preventing sudden death on the athletic field: the emergency action plan. Curr Sports Med Rep 2007;6(2):93–100.

26. Andersen J, Courson RW, Kleiner DM, et al. National Athletic Trainers' Association Position Statement: Emergency Planning in Athletics. J Athl Train 2002;37(1): 99–104.

27. Fu FH, Tjoumakaris FP, Buoncristiani A. Building a sports medicine team. Clin Sports Med 2007;26(2):173–9.

28. Sporer BC, Windt J. Integrated performance support: Facilitating effective and collaborative performance teams. Br J Sports Med 2018;52:1014–5.

29. De Luigi A, Guerrero L. The role of the team physician. In: Mitra R, editor. Principles of rehabilitation medicine. New York: McGraw Hill; 2019. p. 375–87.

30. Herring SA, Kibler WB, Putukian M. Team physician consensus Statement: 2013update. Med Sci Sports Exerc 2013;45(8):1618–22.

31. Dijkstra HP, Pollock N, Chakraverty R, et al. Managing the health of the elite athlete: A new integrated performance health management and coaching model. Br J Sports Med 2014;48:523–31.

32. Lai RY, Krasnow D, Thomas M. Communication between medical practitioners and dancers. J Dance Med Sci 2008;12(2):47–53.

33. Sabo M. Physical therapy rehabilitation strategies for dancers: a qualitative study. J Dance Med Sci 2013;17(1):11–7.

34. Ramkumar PN, Farber J, Arnouk J, et al. Injuries in a professional ballet dance company: A 10 year retrospective study. J Dance Med Sci 2016;20:30–7.

35. Shah S, Weiss DS, Burchette RJ. Injuries in professional modern dancers: incidence, risk factors, and management. J Dance Med Sci 2012;16(1):17–25.
36. Smith PJ, Gerrie BJ, Varner KE, et al. Incidence and Prevalence of Musculoskeletal Injury in Ballet: A Systematic Review. Orthop J Sports Med 2015;3(7). 23259671155592621.
37. Miller C. Dance medicine: current concepts. Phys Med Rehabil Clin N Am 2006; 17(4):803–11, vii.

Concussions in Dancers and Other Performing Artists

Jeffrey A. Russell, PhD, AT, FIADMS[a],*, Lauren McIntyre, ATC[b], Lori Stewart, BPE[c], Tina Wang, MD[d]

KEYWORDS

- Concussion • Head injury • mTBI • Dance • Theater • Circus • Stunt
- Performing arts

KEY POINTS

- Dance and other performing arts are highly physical activities, and performers are subject to head impacts from many sources.
- The amount of scientific literature devoted to concussions in performing arts pales in comparison with that afforded sports concussions.
- Dancers and other performing artists need the same type of timely and sophisticated health care for concussions that traditional athletes receive.
- Performing arts environments require specially designed approaches for managing concussions.

INTRODUCTION

Concussions today receive unparalleled attention; yet, this is virtually exclusive to the context of sports and military applications. The most recent meeting of a premier international consortium on concussion resulted in recommendations devoted entirely to sports.[1] Despite occupational hazards in dance, theater, circus arts, and film/television stunt performance[2–6] (and a large workforce in these artforms), performing arts concussions receive minimal consideration.

Performing arts concussions have virtually no available literature. As a simple demonstration of this, a title keyword search of Pubmed.gov using the string "sport* [ti] AND concussion[ti]" yields nearly 1100 articles. On the other hand, the search "dance*[ti] AND concussion[ti]" returns 3,[5–7] and the search "(theater[ti] OR theater

[a] Ohio University, College of Health Sciences and Professions, School of Applied Health Sciences and Wellness, Grover Center E182, Athens, OH 45701, USA; [b] Harkness Center for Dance Injuries at NYU Langone Health, 614 2nd Avenue, Floor 2, Suite G, New York, NY 10016, USA; [c] Union of British Columbia Performers/ACTRA, 300 – 380 West 2nd Avenue, Vancouver, British Columbia V5Y 1C8, Canada; [d] Loma Linda School of Medicine, Loma Linda VA Hospital, 429 N Central Ave, Upland, CA 91786, USA
* Corresponding author.
E-mail address: jeff.russell@ohio.edu

Phys Med Rehabil Clin N Am 32 (2021) 155–168
https://doi.org/10.1016/j.pmr.2020.09.007
1047-9651/21/© 2020 Elsevier Inc. All rights reserved.

pmr.theclinics.com

[ti]) AND concussion[ti]" returns 1.[4] A similar operation for "film[ti]" offers 1 article: a review in the journal *Neurology* of the motion picture *Concussion* starring actor Will Smith,[8] while concussion searches using "(circus[ti] OR cirque[ti])," "television[ti]," or "stunt*[ti]" yield none.

In light of this scarcity of scholarly literature on the topic of concussions in performing arts, the purposes of this article are to outline the risks of head impact encountered by dancers and other performing artists, establish a case for improved attention to head injuries sustained by artists in dance, theater, circus arts, and film and television stunt work, and transpose current knowledge of sport concussions to prevention and management of this injury in a performance environment. We also hope to engage clinicians' and researchers' interest in caring for and studying the performing arts communities described herein. Although concussion is the injury at hand, the delivery of performing arts health care and clinical research for all injuries is substantially below what is required.

CONCUSSIONS IN DANCE
Prior Research on Dance Concussions

The incidence of concussion in dance is elusive, unlike the well-documented burden of musculoskeletal pain and dysfunction and psychosocial challenges in dance.[9,10] Over the past several years, researchers have begun to identify the risk of concussion in dance. The first known journal article on dance-related concussion was published in 2014.[7] This 5.5-year retrospective case-series identified 11 dance-related concussions of 3011 concussion patients at a large teaching hospital. The patients were 12-year-old to 20-year-old dancers from a variety of styles, including ballet, modern, hip-hop, and acro dance. In 2016, a self-reported survey of ballet and modern dancers between 18 and 71 years old indicated that nearly one-quarter of 153 dancers had sustained a dance-related concussion at some point in their life.[6]

In general, variability in prevalence is seen in the scarce dance concussion literature. Contrasting the study just cited, Harrison and Ruddock-Hudson[11] found that 5.5% of respondents in their sample of 238 collegiate and professional dancers self-reported a history of concussion. In addition, a 2017 study of 480 high school and collegiate dancers found that only 3% had a history of concussion.[12]

The rate of concussion in most sports is higher in competition than in practice.[13,14] In dance, the available literature indicates that concussions occur in class, rehearsal, and performance,[7,15,16] but the relative proportions are unknown. Dancers also may suffer concussions outside of dance or sport-related activities.[7] Thus, continued research is needed to distinguish whether one type of dance activity carries more risk than another.

When considering concussion in dance styles besides modern and ballet, data are even more scant. However, one study identified 2 self-reported concussions in 450 nonprofessional salsa dancers who responded to a survey about their injuries.[17] Although most of these studies suggest that the prevalence of concussion in dance is low, high-quality, prospective epidemiologic studies are needed to investigate the true risk of concussion for dancers across all genres. Furthermore, dancers' often adverse perceptions of health care professionals[18] coupled with a psyche that is reticent to sit out of dance to let injuries heal[19] suggests that predictions of the incidence and prevalence of concussion in dance to date may be deceptively low.

Mechanisms of Dance Concussions

The mechanisms for dance-related concussions can be contact or noncontact in nature. Investigators have reported dance-related concussions due to stunting, diving, flipping, unintentional drops while partnering, slips and falls, direct blows to the head, collisions, whipping the head and neck repeatedly, and head movements combined with high-speed chest or back impacts with the floor or other dancers.[7,15,16]

However, the mechanism of injury in some instances may be elusive. Data point to repetitive, symptomless subconcussive impacts as contributors to functional changes in the brain over time.[20] In addition, it is possible that recurrent head impact exposure could decrease concussion tolerance, meaning a concussion could occur from lower than expected forces.[21,22] One report recounted a dancer sustaining a concussion from repeated forward rolls during a class.[16] The dancer could not identify a specific head impact incident, but developed symptoms afterward. In the case-series of Stein and colleagues,[7] 2 of the concussed dancers were unable to identify a single incident that led to the development of symptoms. One dancer performed several consecutive "diving somersaults" in an acro class and the other was frequently practicing choreography that involved repeatedly whipping her head backward and forward.

Concussion Management in Dancers

Many, if not most, dancers do not have access to a health care practitioner during classes, rehearsals, or performances, so the responsibility for identifying head impacts that may result in a concussion often falls to the teachers, choreographers, directors, or dancers themselves. In addition, concussion symptoms, as distinguished from concussion signs, are internally focused (eg, fatigue, noise sensitivity, fogginess); a dancer must be able to recognize these, know how to communicate the desire to be evaluated for a possible concussion, and select the individual to whom this should be reported.[23]

In light of these factors, awareness of concussion and its management guidelines are critical for the dance community. To begin educating dancers about concussion, the Dance/USA Task Force on Dancer Health wrote an informational paper that presents signs and symptoms, acute management, recovery, and return to dance.[24] However, knowing concussion signs and symptoms may be insufficient to significantly influence management. Studies on concussion knowledge and reporting behaviors, again in a sports context, have shown that concussion knowledge is not necessarily associated with concussion reporting.[25-27] Moreover, in a dance-related study, dancers demonstrated their familiarity with concussions, but their behaviors when confronted with this injury were not aligned with best practice.[6] Beyond educating dancers about signs and symptoms of concussion and empowering them to speak up, they must be taught how to report, or what Warmath and Winterstein[26] call "reporting skill." This may include practicing each step in the reporting process so that it feels comfortable and familiar in the event of a concussion and identifying the appropriate individuals who should receive such reports.

Dancers may behave contrary to their knowledge of proper concussion management due to dance culture and their personalities. It is not uncommon for dancers to continue dancing through pain. Furthermore, dancers process pain differently from most people,[28] and they may not categorize as an "injury" any pain that does not interfere with their ability to dance.[7,19,29] If a dancer is injured, there is pressure to return quickly, especially if the injury occurs around an important performance.[6,16,29] With regard to concussion specifically, 8 of 11 dancers in the case-series of Stein and colleagues[7] continued dancing after a potential concussion mechanism or while experiencing concussion symptoms. McIntyre and Liederbach[6] reported that 19% of respondents to their online survey self-reported dancing while knowingly concussed. These investigators also identified the most common reason that dancers in their study did not report a concussion: the dancers "didn't think it was serious enough." Similar responses are seen in traditional athletes, suggesting that 50% or more of concussion symptoms are hidden by injured individuals.[26,30,31]

Identifying and managing a concussion promptly is critical, as continuing to dance through a concussion may lead to a prolonged recovery.[32] In a study of 97 collegiate athletes, the recovery times between those with immediate versus delayed management of concussion were compared. On average, those who delayed their post-concussion removal from activity experienced approximately 5 additional days of recovery time.[32] Although dance has not received such research attention, a similar result was found in a pair of dance concussion case studies.[15] Two female dancers in the same conservatory level hit one another's heads during a rehearsal. One of the dancers was immediately removed from activity and instructed to visit the staff athletic trainer for care. The second dancer finished rehearsal and took a 2-hour dance class the following day before seeing the athletic trainer. Both dancers were confirmed to have concussions by the athletic trainer and campus physician. The dancer who was immediately removed from activity returned to dance in 8 days, whereas the dancer with delayed management returned in 13 days.

Overall, the limited peer-reviewed publications on dance concussion and the experiences of dance medicine clinicians suggest that dancers are exposed to concussion risk. Sustaining a concussion is neither infrequent nor inconsequential for dancers. Future research should target sound epidemiology of this injury and barriers to concussion reporting in dance. In addition, dance medicine practitioners should develop strategies to create a culture of proper concussion management.

CONCUSSIONS IN THEATER, CIRCUS ARTS, AND FILM/TELEVISION
Prior Research on Theater and Circus Arts

To our knowledge there are 6 primary research articles about theater or circus injuries related to head impacts. Only 1 study is singularly devoted to this topic; it reported survey results of head impacts and concussion management in theater personnel.[4] The lifetime prevalence of receiving at least 1 theater-related head impact was 67%, with 77% of those participants reporting 3 or more impacts and 39% reporting more than 5. Seventy percent of the sample reported having received a head impact resulting in concussion-like symptoms and continuing to participate in their theater work. Only approximately one-third of individuals with symptoms reported their injury to a health care professional; of those, 70% were diagnosed with a concussion. This suggests that in theater personnel there is a high prevalence of concussions as a result of head impacts and that a cultural shift emphasizing head injury reporting is needed.

Two of the 6 articles reported concurrent head and neck injuries, but did not provide further clinical categorization.[33,34] One survey found no head injuries in cirque performers.[35] Another study identified head involvement in 15.2% of accidents in acrobatic styles of theater activities over 17 years,[36] although the investigators did not elaborate about the types of head injuries encountered. Finally, a 5-year study of 1376 Cirque du Soleil performers revealed 7 concussions that each resulted in a time-loss of 15 days or more.[37] Interestingly, the investigators reported concussions under the category "Head and Neck," although such categorization makes capturing the true incidence of concussion impossible. Overall, then, currently available research reveals barriers to ensuring that head injuries in theater and circus are prevented when possible and identified and well-managed when they occur.

Prior Research on Film and Television Stunt Performance

We now focus on an area of performance that may have the greatest discrepancy between likelihood of concussion (high) and volume of concussion research data (virtually none) in all of performing arts. What follows is, to our knowledge, the first attempt to introduce this topic to the scientific literature.

Despite the popularity of stunt sequences and action films, scientific research dedicated to stunt-related concussions, their epidemiology, and how they affect stunt performers longitudinally is nonexistent. Rather, "data" about concussions in this population are reported by the popular media[38–41] and may fail to address the significant morbidity associated with these injuries. The portrayal of concussions sustained by celebrities is often glorified; performers are praised for "toughing it out" when working through their injuries.[42] This tendency, then, ignores most of the industry's performers who experience head injuries.

Because of the paucity of scientific research, addressing concussions in film/television, one of the most influential industries in modern global society, requires reliance on those inside the industry. Underreporting of injuries by stunt performers is strongly aligned with the foundational "cowboy culture" woven throughout stunt-performing communities. Although health and safety awareness and reporting are slowly improving, a research-based approach is needed to better understand the epidemiology of concussion in stunt performance, the mechanisms of injury, and the long-term sequelae.

The 2 known studies of concussion in stunt performance, one a doctoral thesis and the other an organizational whitepaper, were performed in Canada (a country with a large film-making community that produces motion pictures and television for worldwide distribution, especially in North America). The dissertation study by McMichael[43] involving 55 respondents revealed that 82% of stunt performers surveyed reported at least 1 concussion in their career. Fifty-three percent reported at least 1 episode of unconsciousness from a head impact, and there was a mean of 5 concussions per respondent. This is not surprising, although stunt performers hesitate to report head injuries and they lack an appropriate concussion management system.

In addition, this research indicated that stunt performers who experience more lifetime concussions score worse on the cognitive and quality-of-life measures of the Immediate Post-Concussion Assessment and Cognitive Test (ImPACT). This suggests that these artists, clearly at risk for multiple head impacts throughout their careers, are susceptible to long-term decrements in brain function and quality of life. The process of aging may highlight these decreases further.[43]

In 2012, the Actsafe Safety Association in Vancouver, Canada, commissioned a study of British Columbia stunt performers that yielded 188 responses.[44] This research underscored the pervasiveness of underreporting by the artists. By comparing their data with data from the aforementioned PhD dissertation,[43] they revealed a wide difference in concussion reporting frequency between the 2 studies. Remarkably, only 3 of an estimated 400 stunt performers in British Columbia reported concussions to and received compensation from WorkSafeBC between 2002 and 2011, a stark difference from McMichael's[43] 80% prevalence of at least one concussion.

The primary rationale given by respondents in this survey for not reporting injuries was a lack of recognition of the severity of the injuries.[44] Other reasons offered by the performers included perceiving that injuries are part of their job, believing that reporting injuries adversely affects future employment opportunities, and desiring to avoid the bureaucracy of workers' compensation regulatory agencies. These real-world considerations are obstacles to seeking appropriate health care.

Management of Concussion on TV/Film Sets

Historically, recognition and management of concussions on film sets have been poor, particularly in comparison with the sizable advancements in concussion care in sports. The rigor of the stunt industry and the demands on stunt performers' bodies strongly suggests that these performing artists are athletes. These "industrial athletes" typically maintain high levels of physical fitness as they enter stunt work from a variety of sports, including gymnastics, martial arts, dance, diving, climbing, football, hockey, parkour, circus, motocross, and car racing. In spite of the similarities of the participants to traditional athletes, as well as the frequent high-velocity collisions, falls, and related physical requirements of their profession, concerted efforts to provide concussion care lags well behind. Athletic trainers (United States), athletic therapists (Canada), sports medicine physicians, and similarly qualified health care professionals are not employed on-set.

In 2019 the British Columbia Injury Research and Prevention Unit, in consultation with film industry stakeholders, created an industry-specific flowchart[45] to address the unique concussion risks faced by performers. This document, based on a protocol pathway called the Concussion Awareness Training Tool (CATT),[46] addresses concussions occurring in the workplace. It provides an easy-to-follow roadmap for improving the response to and management of any worker suspected of a concussion, including those in the motion picture, television, and live events industries. Applied appropriately, this flowchart—combined with increased training for on-set first aid attendants and emergency medical services personnel—has the potential to improve the recognition and management of concussion in all film industry workers.

Uniqueness and Dangers of Stunt Work and TV/Film Set Environments

Stunt performers work in a unique, fast-paced, high-pressure environment. They are expected to perform at any time of day or night, in restrictive costumes, and often in inherently dangerous settings. They must execute stunts flawlessly on the first "take" (a single attempt of a stunt), with subsequent takes being equally perfect. Stunts performed incorrectly can slow or halt production; the financial consequences of this to the filmmaker can be immense. With thousands, or even hundreds of thousands, of dollars at stake, the pressure for stunt performers to ignore and not report injuries is overwhelming.

Furthermore, stunt performers' employment and, thus, their income, is often sporadic and unpredictable. Being uninjured and otherwise healthy is paramount for performing well and earning a living; therefore, the incentive to hide injuries that could affect their personal livelihood and reputation, apart from the repercussions to the production itself, is high because an injury jeopardizes all future work. When a concussion is suspected, most performers will claim they are "fine" unless they are unconscious or exhibit red flag signs and symptoms.[1,45] Most will participate in subsequent takes and continue working while experiencing concussion symptoms, typically repeating the exact same action that just created their injury.

In the face of these pressures, second impact syndrome (sustaining a second significant head impact before resolution of the first concussion)[20,47] is a rare, but serious, concern. This syndrome is not a universally accepted diagnosis in the concussion management field[48] and is difficult to track and assess.[47] Nonetheless, the severity of its outcome further emphasizes the importance of appropriate concussion protocols for stunt performers, dancers, acrobats, and all other performers in film, television, and live performance.

Concussion risk and inadequate care for stunt performers present substantial challenges. Neurologic compromise may occur, including impaired spatial awareness, attention to detail, reflex timing, proprioception, balance, and memory. The safe execution of stunts requires that all of these neurologic systems be well functioning. The Sport Concussion Assessment Tool version 5 (SCAT5)[49] is recommended for assessment by a qualified health care professional in the stunt context.

Subconcussive head impacts[50] previously discussed in the dance environment may elicit even broader concern for the stunt-performing community. Whiplash mechanisms, also identified as contributors to concussion,[1] are commonplace, as well. They most often occur during falls or fight sequences that require multiple repetitions of the same maneuver; these actions are fundamental techniques for stunt performers working in film. Of particular concern are "head takes" or "head sells" when a performer simulates a reaction to a punch or blow to the head during fight sequences. These movements are small, self-inflicted whiplashes that help make the fake punch or blow look real on camera; the head is snapped quickly in relative proportion to the force and direction of the feigned impact.

Another stunt genre that results in multiple subconcussive blow is falls, whether straightforward falls to the ground or falling off buildings, cliffs, vehicles, and so forth. Performers also are launched into, onto, or through many kinds of surfaces, such as walls, building windows, vehicles, furniture, and the like. The use of mechanical devices like ratchets and air rams increases the velocity and resulting energy of the stunts by flying a performer into a collision with the target object.

Clinical and industry experience suggests that much of the risk to stunt performers' brains is associated with rehearsals rather than with filming on "camera day." In the past 10 years, there has been increased use of pre-visualizations (or, pre-viz) in stunt rehearsals; these may increase a stunt performer's exposure to concussive episodes. In a pre-viz, a stunt coordinator or fight choreographer films rehearsals multiple times from all angles to produce a video proof for the director. Although this process saves time and production costs on the day of shooting, it increases the exposure of stunt performers to several repetitions of full effort stunts. Furthermore, a pre-viz is often filmed after multiple rehearsals within an 8-hour day that are designed to make each stunt "camera-ready." This results in the potential for tens to hundreds of impacts and whiplashes per day.

The careers of typical stunt performers span much longer than those of traditional athletes. These artists frequently enter the stunt profession with a concussion history from prior athletic pursuits. A strong dose-response relationship is seen between duration of football activity and chronic traumatic encephalopathy.[51] The work environment of stunt performers places this community at similar risk, and the length of stunt performers' careers accentuates this concern. Therefore, research with stunt performers must focus on identifying exposures, the forces to which the head is subjected, and ways to ameliorate these.

GENERAL PRINCIPLES OF CONCUSSION CARE FOR PERFORMING ARTS

The management of concussion, or traumatic brain injury (TBI), in performing arts is extrapolated from observational studies in athletes, clinical experience, and consensus guidelines.[1] The principles of management of performing arts–related concussion are similar to those for sport-related concussion with nuances that adjust for the cultural and psychological aspects unique to the performing arts population.

Environmental and Cultural Aspects

Performing arts are demanding disciplines that combine high levels of physical and artistic skill.[9] Performing artists devote their lives to their artform, training from a young age for long hours and often sacrificing other pursuits and interests.[11] The work is rigorous, involving high training loads without rest nor a clearly defined season.[52] These demands are exacerbated by irregular sleep, rehearsal, and performance schedules.[53] Such conditions make performing artists particularly susceptible to injury.[54]

Psychosocial Aspects

Psychosocial issues make reporting and managing performing arts-associated TBI particularly challenging. Performing artists exhibit a high level of psychopathological symptoms compared with the general population.[55] The constant performance-focus promotes maladaptive tendencies like compulsivity, perfectionism, eating disorders, and depression.[55,56] These maladaptive disorders aggravate injuries and compound underreporting of injuries generally[57] and with regard to TBI.[6]

Translation of Sports Concussion Management to Performing Arts

Return to performance protocols

The management of performing arts–related concussions should follow closely the care guidelines for sport-related concussions, while accounting for the bio-psychosocial distinctives specific to the performing arts. Artists should be evaluated by a licensed practitioner familiar with concussion diagnosis and management (eg, primary care physician, athletic trainer) who will determine the extent of TBI and offer guidance on monitoring and management.[58] Artists with persistent symptoms beyond 2 to 3 weeks, multiple concussion history, or uncertain diagnosis of TBI should be referred to a physician with specific expertise in managing concussions (eg, sports medicine specialist, physiatrist, or neurologist).[58]

The timing for return to school, work, rehearsals, and performances should be individualized and based on symptoms and individual clinical course.[59] A graded return to performance protocol advances through the stages presented in **Table 1**. It is important to note that typical concussion evaluations and graduated "return to play" protocols are created with sports jargon (eg, field, game, contest, half). Thus, health care providers working with performing artists must adapt these instruments to accommodate to the artist's particular artistic environment. Artists should remain at each stage

Table 1	
Stages for a graded return to performing arts activity	
Stage 1	Cognitive rest/light stretching (relative rest)
Stage 2	Proprioceptive training Light sub-threshold aerobic activity Dance or barre warm-up Cognitive/Speech therapy Mark class and performance piece
Stage 3	Continue proprioceptive training Start class with 25% effort and participation in daily performing arts routine Continue marking class and performance piece
Stage 4	50% effort and participation in daily performing arts routine Continue marking class and performance piece
Stage 5	Full effort and participation in daily performing arts routine Continue marking performance piece
Stage 6	Rehearsal
Stage 7	Performance

of rehabilitation for no less than 24 hours before advancing to the next level; a minimum of 5 days should pass before consideration of return to full performance.[1]

Initial management should be complete removal from performance for that day's or night's activities[1,58,59] to avoid additional head injury that may lead to second impact syndrome,[60,61] and to provide cognitive and physical rest.[1,59] Cognition is particularly important to performing artists; they must memorize lines or music, engage in complex choreography, focus on technical skills, and learn new material quickly.[62] Artists also may be subject to perturbing environmental factors such as bright stage lights, heavily amplified sound, and special effects such as fog or other disorienting stimuli. In this initial stage, a performer may engage in light stretching.[63] Toward the end of this stage, "marking" (where the artist performs an attenuated version of a performance using mental visualization) is effective and may be used as a prelude to its use throughout the return to performance stages.[64]

Relative rest should be followed by a gradual and progressive return to performance that is individualized at a rate and intensity to avoid symptom exacerbation.[59] Given performing artists' propensity to continue performing despite TBI symptoms,[4] good clinician-patient communication is crucial. Performing artists also should be advised that early aerobic sub-symptom threshold exercise may hasten recovery,[65] whereas noncompliance with return to performance activity before symptom resolution may lead to prolonged continuation of symptoms.[66]

Pharmacologic management
Pharmacologic interventions generally should be avoided; however, a brief period of symptom management with medications may be warranted in consultation with the artist's treating physician. Return to performance should not occur while taking medication. Worsening of symptoms despite judicious medication prescription and appropriate physical and cognitive rest warrants evaluation with advanced imaging for other potential diagnoses and serious complications.[67]

Effectiveness of education and baseline testing
Culture change regarding concussion in performing arts is needed, but the effectiveness of education is controversial. Educational programs in high-risk sports have been associated with increased recognition and acknowledgment of the seriousness of TBI.[68] However, these programs are not likely to change behavior in athletes, a phenomenon that also has been demonstrated with performing artists.[6] Performing artists and athletes alike seem determined to hide symptoms, or not report them, in order to continue performing.[27]

Baseline cognitive testing may encourage cultural change because such assessment analyzes cognitive function before concussion[69] and can provide evidence of concussion-mediated alterations postinjury. Baseline, acute stageside, and follow-up serial assessments also are useful for detecting evolving neurologic emergencies.[70] Baseline evaluations may be particularly helpful for performing artists who exhibit a history of headaches, migraines, and psychiatric conditions that may influence scores. Therefore, capturing these initially is beneficial to the care paradigm.[5,71]

SUMMARY

Although a dearth of performing arts–specific concussion research besets a field of endeavor comprising specialized groups of artist-athletes, undeniable is the risk of head injury to which these individuals are routinely exposed. In an unmitigated contrast to sports, performing arts lack the necessary health care and research attention to concussion occurrence. Dance, theater, and circus all present their participants with concussion exposure, but stunt performers in film and television may be at the highest risk of this injury among artists, especially for chronic sequelae. Thus, performing arts represent needful opportunities for engagement by clinicians and researchers alike.

CLINICS CARE POINTS

- Recognizing the risk of concussion in performing arts is an important prelude to the prompt identification and management of this injury in performers.
- The identification of concussion in performing artists is challenging, as repetitive, symptomless, subconcussive impacts may be long-term contributors.
- Baseline, acute stageside, and follow-up serial assessments are useful for detecting evolving neurologic deficits or emergencies.
- Management principles for performing arts–related concussion are similar to those for sport-related concussion, with nuances that adjust for cultural and psychological aspects unique to the performing arts population. These include rigorous, training loads, maladaptive tendencies, special cognitive requirements, and a propensity for non-compliance.
- Concussion-mediated alterations post-injury may promote cultural change through education of artists, directors, and other personnel.

CONFLICT OF INTEREST

None of the authors have conflicts of interest to disclose in connection with the topic of this paper.

REFERENCES

1. McCrory P, Meeuwisse W, Dvořák J, et al. Consensus statement on concussion in sport: the 5th International Conference on Concussion in Sport held in Berlin, October 2016. Br J Sports Med 2017;51(11):838–47.
2. Rossol M. The health and safety guide for film, TV, and theater. New York: Allworth Press; 2011.
3. Rossol M, Hinkamp D. Hazards in the theater. Occup Med 2001;16(4):595–608.
4. Russell JA, Daniell BM. Concussion in theater: a cross-sectional survey of prevalence and management in actors and theater technicians. J Occup Environ Med 2018;60(3):205–10.
5. McIntyre L, Campo M. Descriptive values for dancers on baseline concussion tools. J Athl Train 2017;52(11):1035–40.
6. McIntyre L, Liederbach M. Concussion knowledge and behaviors in a sample of the dance community. J Dance Med Sci 2016;20(2):79–88.
7. Stein CJ, Kinney SA, McCrystal T, et al. Dance-related concussion: a case series. J Dance Med Sci 2014;18(2):53–61.
8. Siegler JE, Wesley SF. Right brain: concussion (film): review and historical context. Neurology 2016;87(14):e155–8. https://doi.org/10.1212/WNL. 0000000000003174.
9. Koutedakis Y, Jamurtas A. The dancer as a performing athlete: physiological considerations. Sports Med 2004;34(10):651–61.
10. Liederbach M, Dilgen FE, Rose DJ. Incidence of anterior cruciate ligament injuries among elite ballet and modern dancers: a 5-year prospective study. Am J Sports Med 2008;36(9):1779–88.

11. Harrison C, Ruddock-Hudson M. Perceptions of pain, injury, and transition-retirement: the experiences of professional dancers. J Dance Med Sci 2017; 21(2):43–52.

12. Yau RK, Golightly YM, Richardson DB, et al. Potential predictors of injury among pre-professional ballet and contemporary dancers. J Dance Med Sci 2017;21(2): 53–63.

13. Kerr Z, Chandran A, Nedimyer A, et al. Concussion incidence and trends in 20 high school sports. Pediatrics 2019;144(5):e20192180.

14. Putukian M, D'Alonzo B, Campbell-McGovern C, et al. The Ivy League-Big Ten epidemiology of concussion study: a report on methods and first findings. Am J Sports Med 2019;47(5):1236–47.

15. McIntyre L. Concussion recovery in two dancers: a case study. J Athl Train 2019; 54(6s):S219–20.

16. Kish R, Koutures C. The invisible injury: supporting the recovery of dancers with concussions. J Phys Educ Recreat Dance 2016;87(8):27–32.

17. Domene PA, Stanley M, Skamagki G. Injury surveillance of nonprofessional salsa dance. J Phys Act Health 2018;15(10):774–80.

18. Wang TJ, Russell JA. A tenuous pas de deux: examining university dancers' access to and satisfaction with healthcare delivery. Med Probl Perform Art 2018; 33(2):111–7.

19. Thomas H, Tarr J. Dancers' perceptions of pain and injury: positive and negative effects. J Dance Med Sci 2009;13(2):51–9.

20. Stemper B, Shah A, Harezlak J, et al. Exposure in college football following an NCAA rule change to eliminate two-a-day preseason practices: a study from the NCAA-DoD CARE Consortium. Ann Biomed Eng 2019;47(10):2073–85.

21. Stemper B, Shah A, Harezlak J, et al. Comparison of head impact exposure between concussed football athletes and matched controls: evidence for a possible second mechanism of sport-related concussion. Ann Biomed Eng 2019;47(10): 2057–72.

22. Rowson S, Campolettano E, Duma S, et al. Accounting for variance in concussion tolerance between individuals: comparing head accelerations between concussed and physically matched control subjects. Ann Biomed Eng 2019;47: 2048–56.

23. Corman S, Adame B, Tsai J, et al. Socioecological influences on concussion reporting by NCAA Division 1 athletes in high-risk sports. PLoS One 2019;14(5): e0215424.

24. Dance/USA Task Force on Dancer Health. Tips on concussion for dancers. Dance USA Informational Papers. 2019. Available at: https://dance-usa.s3.amazonaws. com/page_uploads/Concussion.10.26.15.pdf. Accessed May 18, 2020.

25. Kroshus E, Baugh C, Daneshvar D, et al. Concussion reporting intention: a valuable metric for predicting reporting behavior and evaluating concussion education. Clin J Sport Med 2015;25(3):243–7.

26. Warmath D, Winterstein AP. Reporting skill: the missing ingredient in concussion reporting intention assessment. Sports Health 2019;11(5):416–24.

27. Beidler E, Bretzin A, Hanock C, et al. Sport-related concussion: knowledge and reporting behaviors among collegiate club-sport athletes. J Athl Train 2018; 53(9):866–72.

28. Tajet-Foxell B, Rose FD. Pain and pain tolerance in professional ballet dancers. Br J Sports Med 1995;29(1):31–4.

29. Anderson R, Hanrahan S. Dancing in pain: pain appraisal and coping in dancers. J Dance Med Sci 2008;12(1):9–16.

30. Chrisman S, Quitiquit C, Rivara F. Qualitative study of barriers to concussive symptom reporting in high school athletics. J Adolesc Health 2013;52(3):330–5.

31. McCrea M, Hammeke T, Olsen G, et al. Unreported concussion in high school football players: implications for prevention. Clin J Sport Med 2004;14(1):13–7.

32. Asken B, McCrea M, Clugston J, et al. "Playing through it": delayed reporting and removal from athletic activity after concussion predicts prolonged recovery. J Athl Train 2016;51(4):329–35.

33. Evans RW, Evans RI, Carvajal S, et al. A survey of injuries among Broadway performers. Am J Public Health 1996;86(1):77–80.

34. Evans RW, Evans RI, Carvajal S. Survey of injuries among West End performers. Occup Environ Med 1998;55(9):585–93.

35. Long AS, Ambegaonkar JP, Fahringer PM. Injury reporting rates and injury concealment patterns differ between high-school cirque performers and basketball players. Med Probl Perform Art 2011;26(4):200–5.

36. Wanke EM, McCormack M, Koch F, et al. Acute injuries in student circus artists with regard to gender specific differences. Asian J Sports Med 2012;3(3):153–60.

37. Shrier I, Meeuwisse WH, Matheson GO, et al. Injury patterns and injury rates in the circus arts: an analysis of 5 years of data from Cirque du Soleil. Am J Sports Med 2009;37(6):1143–9. https://doi.org/10.1177/0363546508331138.

38. Robinson K. 9 celebrities who have suffered from concussions: who knew acting and singing could be such a dangerous job? EverydayHealth.com. 2018. Available at: https://www.everydayhealth.com/neurology/living-with/celebrities-who-have-concussions/. Accessed May 13, 2020.

39. Broadway. com. Bret Michaels settles court case after 2009 Tony Awards injury. 2012. Available at: https://www.broadway.com/buzz/161883/bret-michaels-settles-court-case-after-2009-tony-awards-injury/. Accessed May 18, 2020.

40. Sciarpelletti L. Concussions go ignored on film sets, says Vancouver stunt performer. 2019. Available at: https://www.cbc.ca/news/canada/british-columbia/stunt-film-set-performer-supergirl-xmen-lori-stewart-1.5194081. Accessed February 5, 2020.

41. Robb D. OSHA fines 'MacGyver' producers for accident that left stuntman badly injured. Deadline. 2019. Available at: https://deadline.com/2019/02/macgyver-stuntman-accident-osha-fines-producers-1202560583/. Accessed February 20, 2019.

42. Rose S. Film stunts under scrutiny after deaths and serious injuries. The Guardian. 2019. Available at: http://www.theguardian.com/film/2019/jul/26/film-stunts-under-scrutiny-after-deaths-and-serious-injuries. Accessed May 13, 2020.

43. McMichael LP. The effects of concussions in stunt performers (Doctoral Dissertation). Santa Barbara, California: Fielding Graduate University; 2007.

44. Quirke B. Stunt related injuries in the motion picture and film industry: a literature review. Vancouver (Canada): Actsafe Safety Association; 2012.

45. British Columbia Injury Research and Prevention Unit. Concussion awareness, response, and management flowchart. Vancouver (Canada): Actsafe Safety Association; 2019. Available at: https://www.actsafe.ca/topic/concussion/concussion-awareness-response-and-management-flowchart/. Accessed May 18, 2020.

46. Concussion Awareness Training Tool. CATT Flipcard, Adults. 2019. Available at: https://cattonline.com/wp-content/uploads/2019/09/CATT-Flip-Card-V1-June-2019-Adults-EN-web.pdf. Accessed May 18, 2020.

47. Engelhardt J, Brauge D, Loiseau H. Second impact syndrome. Myth or reality? Neurochirurgie 2020. https://doi.org/10.1016/j.neuchi.2019.12.007.

48. McLendon LA, Kralik SF, Grayson PA, et al. The controversial second impact syndrome: a review of the literature. Pediatr Neurol 2016;62:9–17.
49. BMJ Publishing Group Ltd. Sport concussion assessment tool - 5th edition. Br J Sports Med 2017;51(11):851–8.
50. Bailes JE, Petraglia AL, Omalu BI, et al. Role of subconcussion in repetitive mild traumatic brain injury. J Neurosurg 2013;119(5):1235–45.
51. Mez J, Daneshvar DH, Abdolmohammadi B, et al. Duration of American football play and chronic traumatic encephalopathy. Ann Neurol 2020;87(1):116–31.
52. Twitchett E, Angioi M, Koutedakis Y, et al. The demands of a working day among female professional ballet dancers. J Dance Med Sci 2010;14(4):127–32.
53. Jeffries AC, Wallace L, Coutts AJ. Quantifying training loads in contemporary dance. Int J Sports Physiol Perform 2017;12(6):796–802.
54. Kenny SJ, Palacios-Derflingher L, Shi Q, et al. Association between previous injury and risk factors for future injury in preprofessional ballet and contemporary dancers. Clin J Sport Med 2019;29(3):209–17.
55. van Staden A, Myburgh CPH, Poggenpoel M. A psycho-educational model to enhance the self-development and mental health of classical dancers. J Dance Med Sci 2009;13(1):20–8.
56. Wainwright SP, Williams C, Turner BS. Fractured identities: injury and the balletic body. Health (London) 2005;9(1):49–66.
57. Mainwaring LM, Finney C. Psychological risk factors and outcomes of dance injury: a systematic review. J Dance Med Sci 2017;21(3):87–96.
58. Harmon KG, Drezner JA, Gammons M, et al. American Medical Society for Sports Medicine position statement on concussion in sport. Br J Sports Med 2013;47(1): 15–26.
59. Lumba-Brown A, Yeates KO, Sarmiento K, et al. Centers for Disease Control and Prevention guideline on the diagnosis and management of mild traumatic brain injury among children. JAMA Pediatr 2018;172(11):e182853.
60. Yumul JN, McKinlay A. Do multiple concussions lead to cumulative cognitive deficits? A literature review. PM R 2016;8(11):1097–103.
61. Kucera KL, Yau RK, Register-Mihalik J, et al. Traumatic brain and spinal cord fatalities among high school and college football players — United States, 2005–2014. MMWR Morb Mortal Wkly Rep 2017;65(52):1465–9.
62. Stevens CJ, Vincs K, deLahunta S, et al. Long-term memory for contemporary dance is distributed and collaborative. Acta Psychol (Amst) 2019;194:17–27.
63. Sinnott AM, Elbin RJ, Collins MW, et al. Persistent vestibular-ocular impairment following concussion in adolescents. J Sci Med Sport 2019;22(12):1292–7.
64. Moran A, Guillot A, MacIntyre T, et al. Re-imagining motor imagery: Building bridges between cognitive neuroscience and sport psychology: Re-imagining motor imagery. Br J Psychol 2012;103(2):224–47.
65. Willer BS, Haider MN, Bezherano I, et al. Comparison of rest to aerobic exercise and placebo-like treatment of acute sport-related concussion in male and female adolescents. Arch Phys Med Rehabil 2019;100(12):2267–75.
66. Hiploylee C, Dufort PA, Davis HS, et al. Longitudinal study of postconcussion syndrome: not everyone recovers. J Neurotrauma 2017;34(8):1511–23.
67. de la Tremblaye PB, O'Neil DA, LaPorte MJ, et al. Elucidating opportunities and pitfalls in the treatment of experimental traumatic brain injury to optimize and facilitate clinical translation. Neurosci Biobehav Rev 2018;85:160–75.
68. Institute of Medicine, National Research Council. Sports-related concussions in youth: improving the science, changing the culture. Washington, DC: The

National Academies Press; 2014. Available at: http://www.ncbi.nlm.nih.gov/books/NBK169016/. Accessed December 21, 2019.

69. Putukian M. The acute symptoms of sport-related concussion: diagnosis and on-field management. Clin Sports Med 2011;30(1):49–61, viii.

70. Podell K, Presley C, Derman H. Sideline sports concussion assessment. Neurol Clin 2017;35(3):435–50.

71. Cottle JE, Hall EE, Patel K, et al. Concussion baseline testing: preexisting factors, symptoms, and neurocognitive performance. J Athl Train 2017;52(2):77–81.

Dry Needling and Acupuncture in Treatment of Dance-Related Injuries, MD, and PT Perspectives

Amanda M. Blackmon, PT, DPT[a,b,c,d,*], Lauren Elson, MD[e,f,1]

KEYWORDS

- Acupuncture • Neurofunctional acupuncture • Dry needling • Trigger point
- Myofascial pain • Musculoskeletal pain • Complementary medicine

KEY POINTS

- Trigger points are a source of pain and dysfunction for dancers.
- Health care practitioners can augment their care of the dancer with needling techniques.
- Stimulation of local tissue with a needle can have both local and systemic pain relieving effects.
- Needling changes the local chemical milieu and may improve tissue healing.
- Dry needling and acupuncture can be safe and effective techniques for treating musculo-skeletal pain in dancers.

ACUPUNCTURE

Acupuncture is the stimulation of anatomic, neuroreactive points on the body with needles to affect change. Documents from 100 BCE demonstrate its use in China, and it later spread to other Asian countries. It eventually lost status in China but was brought to Europe by Portuguese missionaries in the sixteenth century.[1] Its first use in the United States was recorded in 1826 when a US Navy surgeon used it to treat back pain. Acupuncture became popularized in the United States in 1971 when New York Times reporter James Reston wrote about doctors in China using needles to

[a] Department of Physical Therapy, College of Health Professions, Mercer University, Atlanta, GA, USA; [b] Myopain Seminars, Atlanta Ballet; [c] Atlanta Dance Medicine, Atlanta, GA, USA; [d] MandyDancePT, LLC, Atlanta, GA, USA; [e] Spaulding Rehabilitation, Boston, MA, USA; [f] Physical Medicine and Rehabilitation, Harvard Medical School, Boston, MA, USA
[1] Present address: 65 Walnut St, Wellesley, MA, 02481.
* Corresponding author. 601 Houze Way, Roswell, GA 30076.
E-mail address: MandyDancePT@gmail.com
Twitter: @mandydancePT (A.M.B.); @laurenelsonMD (L.E.)

Phys Med Rehabil Clin N Am 32 (2021) 169–183
https://doi.org/10.1016/j.pmr.2020.08.005
1047-9651/21/© 2020 Elsevier Inc. All rights reserved.
pmr.theclinics.com

ease his pain after surgery.[2] Today, practitioners of acupuncture may incorporate techniques from China, Japan, and Korea among others.

Although the intricacies of the various systems are different, including restoring imbalances of the flow of qi ("life force" or energy flow), restoring yin/yang energy balance, and balancing organ-based channels of energy, the effects on the body can be explained by tangible science. It is known that needles influence subtle electrical flow in multiple ways. There is a thermoelectric phenomenon where the temperature gradient from the tip is warmer and cooler at the handle causing the tip to have a slight positive charge. The metal itself creates a small electromagnetic effect, and 2 to 3 microamperes of energy is generated. Manipulation of the needle can increase positive ion attraction, generating a current up to 10 to 15 microamperes.[3] Manipulation can include pistoning, twisting, and running electric current between the needles, also known as electroacupuncture.

Electroacupuncture has been found to have specific effects on neurotransmitters.[4] Low-frequency versus high-frequency electroacupuncture selectively induces the release of enkephalins and dynorphins. For patients with inflammatory conditions, cotreatment with acupuncture and nonsteroidal antiinflammatory drugs seems to be synergistic, as expression of COX-1 and COX-2 is inhibited by 2 Hz treatment with electroacupuncture.[5] Multiple organs generate discrete electric fields and may transmit this to limbs via fascia and interstitial fluid. Transmission of electroionic charge between acupuncture points along fascial planes has been demonstrated, which may explain the energy lines or meridians that are often discussed in traditional forms of acupuncture. The influence of acupuncture on the mu opioid and serotonin receptors affects systems in the body from insulin secretion to potentiation of the effects of endogenous opioids. It seems that the analgesic effects of acupuncture involve supraspinal and spinal mechanisms via its effects on the serotonergic and noradrenergic receptors in the spinal cord.[6]

Acupuncture influences the release, synthesis, reuptake, and degradation of central neurotransmitters/modulators, including serotonin, noradrenalin, dopamine, acetylcholine, substance P, prostaglandin, cholecystokinin octapeptide (CCK-8), somatostatin, and neurotrophic factors. It enhances the activity of the endogenous opioid peptides and inhibitory amino acids. Acupuncture also attenuates the activity of the noradrenalin and excitatory amino acids and regulates the expression and function of the corresponding receptors.[7] Animal models of acupuncture needling demonstrate activation of local satellite (stem) cells 72 hours after needling.[8] Acupuncture improves tissue perfusion by improving vasomotor control and can improve strength by removing motor inhibition. It can influence tissue healing, cell metabolism, tissue remodeling, and adhesions by improving tissue trophism. It works to decrease pain perception by influencing both nociceptive and central pain neuromodulators[9]

Because of its ability to affect multiple systems within the body, acupuncture is an ideal mode of holistic treatment. It can modulate chemical reactions occurring within local tissues, while at the same time affect the regulation of the central nervous system, thus influencing the experience of the recipient. Although acupuncture may not be able to "fix" pathologies within the body, it can optimize the function and resiliency of the body by affecting the nervous system.

The acupuncture described in this article is based on neurofunctional acupuncture.[10] It involves "the stimulation of neurofunctional sites for the therapeutic purpose of modulating abnormal activity of the nervous system and/or the endocrine, exocrine and immune systems, in pain syndromes, functional problems, and any diseases in which these modulatory mechanisms are available." Neuromodulation occurs at multiple levels, including the peripheral nerves, spinal cord, brain stem, brain, and cerebellum. This system is mechanism based, not disease based, with the therapeutic goals and treatment targets based on the neurologic dysfunctions contributing to the clinical presentation.[10] This holistic approach lends itself to treatment of artists in that it can address complex psychosocial factors that contribute to the patient's experience of symptoms. When a dancer is injured, it is rarely an isolated tissue-level event. Besides local tissue disruption and inflammation, the peripheral nervous system and spinal cord are affected. The stress of having an injury can enhance fear, anxiety, and uncertainty, especially in artists who depend on elite physical function for their careers. In this increased state of stress, the sympathetic nervous system can be overly activated and can contribute to mood swings, slow tissue healing, and increased infection susceptibility. Reflex responses and neurotransmission may be altered. In these situations, acupuncture can affect symptoms, by acting both regionally and systemically. Acupuncture has been shown to modulate responses in the hypothalamus, amygdala,[11] and sensorimotor cortex.[12] In order to treat this neurofunctional dysregulation, results are often optimized with several weeks of treatment.

DRY NEEDLING

Dry needling is "a skilled intervention that uses a thin filiform needle to penetrate the skin and stimulate underlying myofascial trigger points, muscular, and connective tissues for the management of neuromusculoskeletal pain and movement impairments," according to the American Physical Therapy Association.[13] Other professions that use dry needling define the technique similarly. There is debate among medical professionals regarding the similarities between dry needling and acupuncture. More than 90% of the traditional 360 traditional acupuncture points were found to correspond to myofascial trigger points and many others correspond to superficial nerves, neuromuscular junctions, and the entheses between ligament or tendon and bone.[14] Although original studies explain the science of acupuncture, the mechanisms are likely similar to those that facilitate change in dry needling, and some of the methods used in the studies could be regarded as either. Both the dry needling and the acupuncture communities draw on the same literature surrounding the microcellular milieu responsible for the understanding of trigger points.[15] Similarly, Dr Karl Lewit described the "needle effect" on multiple tissues throughout the body in 1979. Some of these were superficial techniques, and others were "deep needling," similar to trigger point dry needling as we call it today.[16] The same needles are used with both techniques, and many similar conditions may be treated. There are hundreds of acupuncture systems and approaches and not all can be lumped into one comparative group. Similarly, there are multiple training programs and methodologies for dry needling. For the purposes of simplicity and accuracy, and based on the training of the authors, the techniques discussed primarily refer to trigger point dry needling, which targets myofascial trigger points in muscle tissue.[17]

MYOFASCIAL TRIGGER POINTS

Trigger point dry needling is based on the work of Drs Janet Travell and David Simons and has been expanded on by others.[18–20] Historically, trigger points were treated by injection of various substances using a hypodermic needle. Current research demonstrates that dry needling, the use of a small filiform needle, is as effective or more effective than trigger point injections, without the potential side effects that may occur with medications commonly used with trigger point injections.[21]

Myofascial trigger points are common and may be overlooked as a cause of both acute and chronic pain.[22] A myofascial trigger point is a discrete and palpable nodule within a taut band of muscle that is exquisitely tender with mechanical stimulation.[20] The pain from a myofascial trigger point may remain local or may refer to a different and remote part of the body. Active trigger points reproduce local and referred pain patterns that are recognizable by patients as their familiar pain. Active and latent trigger points share common features: local pain with palpation, referred pain to a distant or remote region, range of motion restrictions, muscle inhibition, and changes in muscle activation patterns and motor control.[23] Both may also feature autonomic phenomena such at lacrimation, sweating, piloerection, etc.[17(p244)] Latent trigger points are different in that they will not produce spontaneous and familiar pain. In addition, the latent trigger points will have a lower pain intensity, smaller referred pain areas, and will feature less cutaneous and subcutaneous sensitivity than their active counterparts.[24] Trigger points may develop in muscle for a variety of reasons, including, but not limited to, trauma, concentric muscle overload, eccentric muscle overload, prolonged postural overload, and repetitive low-load muscle activity.[20] With muscle overload, an energy crisis occurs. Blood flow to the muscle fibers is restricted, causing a back-up or retrograde blow blow. This results in ischemia, decreased oxygenation to the tissue, and a lowering of pH, resulting in an acidic environment. The hypoxia also triggers an increase in acetylcholine (ACh) at the motor end plate.[25] The acidic environment leads to a chemical cascade that will change thresholds and permeability of specific nociceptors, including transient receptor potential vanilloid and acid-sensing ion channels.[26] Concentrations of specific nociceptive chemicals are higher inside a myofascial trigger point, including adenosine triphosphate, bradykinin, 5-hydroxytryptamine, serotonin, prostaglandins, calcitonin gene-related peptide (CGRP), and potassium.[15] It is hypothesized that there are also higher levels of acetylcholine and glutamate, with lowered concentrations of acetylcholinesterase (ACh-esterase). Electrical activity is increased near a trigger point, resulting in motor endplate noise.[27] Increased motor end plate noise indicates that the muscle tissue is never completely relaxing.

There is a "needle effect" with any insertion of a needle into the tissue, which may explain some of the overlap between acupuncture and dry needling results. Trigger point dry needling aims to specifically elicit a localized twitch response (LTR). The LTR is an involuntary spinal cord reflex of muscle fibers in a taut band after a trigger point is stimulated with a solid needle, an injection needle, or a snapping palpation.[21,28] Evidence shows that the LTR can decrease or eliminate endplate noise associated with trigger points, suggesting a deactivation of the trigger point.[28] In addition, eliciting the LTR seems to decrease the concentration of nociceptive chemicals typically found in the immediate milieu of active trigger points.[15] Both the decrease in endplate noise and the decrease in chemicals such as substance P and CGRP may explain the decrease in pain seen clinically after deep dry needling.[15] There is debate in the literature regarding the need to obtain one or many LTRs to achieve positive clinical outcomes. Dommerholt and Fernandez-de-las-Penas[17] acknowledge that many studies arguing against the need for LTRs do not resemble clinical practice in their study design.

CLINICAL EXAMPLES AND APPLICATION

Trigger points may result in impairments including pain, range of motion restrictions, muscle inhibition, increased muscle tone, and changes in muscle activation patterns and motor control.[23] These impairments may be addressed by treating trigger points with dry needling. Referred pain patterns from trigger points may also mimic other musculoskeletal and nerve pathologies and injuries, especially in a dancer population.

For example, a dancer collides with another dancer and her shin develops a large hematoma. The hematoma is painful, but resolves after a normal healing period of 7 to 10 days. However, the dancer begins experiencing anterior ankle and great toe pain with no known trauma or injury to the area. It is possible that the trauma to the shin caused trigger points to develop in the anterior tibialis muscle, which refers directly to the anterior ankle and great toe (**Fig. 1**). Thus, by treating the trigger points in the anterior tibialis, the pain is resolved. Acupuncture could also be added to facilitate healing of the region. Techniques to improve regional blood flow could be used to help the hematoma resolve.

Inhibition of key muscles that provide support or stability may also interfere with symptoms. For example, when the gluteus medius is impaired, there may be abnormal stresses placed on proximal or distal structures.[29] Therefore, one needs to identify and treat trigger points in the kinetic chain but possibly quite far from the painful region. In female athletes with patellofemoral pain syndrome, function and pressure pain threshold were reduced more in subjects receiving dry needling of the gluteus medius and quadratus lumborum (QL) in addition to standardized exercises.[30]

Similarly, there are "key" muscles that practitioners must keep in mind when evaluating a dancer with low back pain, both with and without a radicular pain pattern. The QL is one of these key muscles, as it can mimic a lateral shift in the lumbar spine, may appear as a lumbar scoliotic curvature, and may contribute to a functional leg length discrepancy. In addition, primary trigger points in the QL may cause inhibition and weakness in the gluteal muscles, causing decreased ability to stabilize the hip and pelvic girdle of the ipsilateral side. Therefore, treating the QL first may also help to address additional impairments in the patient's presentation. Other muscles that may be important in the examination of a patient with nonspecific low back pain include the abdominals, the adductors, the lumbar multifidi, and paraspinals, among others.[17,31]

In a dancer presenting with more sciatic nerve or discogenic pain, trigger points should also be considered. For example, according to Travell, the gluteus minimus muscle's referral pattern travels down the posterior and lateral aspect of the thigh, leg, and into the foot[19] (**Fig. 2**). This pattern may mimic a radiculopathy, but the patient may not present with other typical findings of an L4/5 disc herniation: changes in dermatomes, myotomes, reflexes, etc. In addition to these points, an acupuncturist may needle at the spinal segment that correlates with the referred symptoms to modulate the neural response. In addition, trigger points in the deep external rotators of the hip (piriformis, gemelli superior and inferior, obturator internus and externus, and quadratus femoris) may cause shortening of these muscles, limited internal rotation of the hip, and a pain pattern consistent with "piriformis syndrome." Because of muscle length effects, this patient may also present as positive for typical special tests for piriformis syndrome. Clinically, treating the deep rotators should resolve both pain and range of motion restrictions. When dancers present with anterior hip pain, in the setting of decreased external rotation and gluteal trigger points, release of the trigger points is often an effective first step in reducing pain and facilitating recruitment of the muscles for neuromuscular retraining and pelvic stabilization.

Dancers often present with complaints of foot pain; stress fractures/stress reactions should always be considered as a source of symptoms, as stress injuries are more common in this population.[32,33] However, trigger points should also be included in the differential diagnosis. For example, the soleus refers directly to the plantar surface of the calcaneus and may mimic a calcaneal stress fracture (**Fig. 3**). In addition, if trigger points in the soleus are causing muscle shortening, the dancer may also present with limited dorsiflexion and changes in the biomechanics for plié, jumping, and

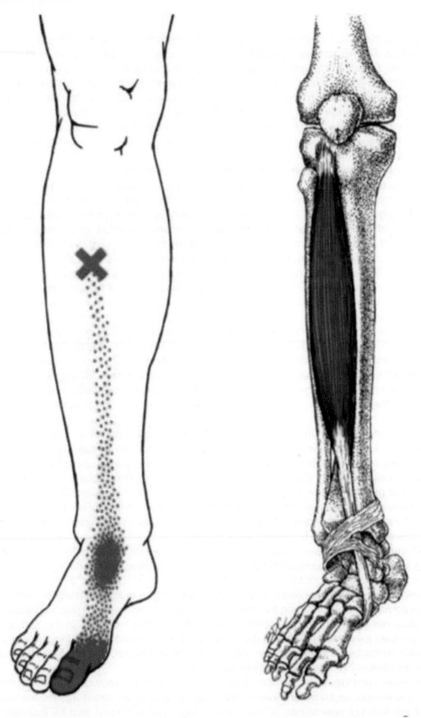

Fig. 1. Tibialis anterior muscle referral pattern. (*From* Donnelly JM, Fernande-de las-Penas C, Finnegan M, et al, eds. Travell, Simons & Simons' Myofascial Pain and Dysfunction. 3rd ed. Philadelphia, PA: Wolters Kluwer;2019:701; with permission.)

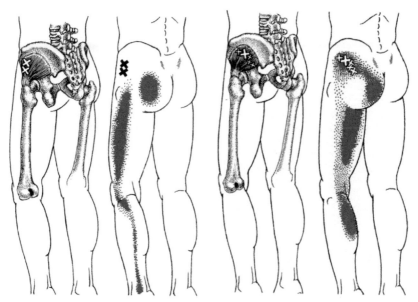

Fig. 2. Gluteus minimus pain referral pattern. (*From* Donnelly JM, Fernande-de las-Penas C, Finnegan M, et al, eds. Travell, Simons & Simons' Myofascial Pain and Dysfunction. 3rd ed. Philadelphia, PA: Wolters Kluwer;2019:679; with permission.)

landing. Other common sites for stress responses include the anterior tibia, distal fibula, and metatarsals.[33] All of these may have trigger points as contributing factors to the pain presentation: tibialis anterior, fibularis muscles, extensor digitorum longus and brevis, extensor hallucis longus and brevis, and plantar and dorsal interossei, among others (**Fig. 4**).

Dancers are often diagnosed with plantar fasciitis when presenting with pain in the arch of the foot.[34] In addition to traditional treatments, the practitioner should consider a group of muscles that may be related to this pain presentation, especially in a dancer who has recently increased jumping volume. Gastrocnemius should be examined first, as it refers directly to the arch and may also limit dorsiflexion range of motion.[19] Other muscles to consider include flexor digitorum longus, quadratus plantae (flexor accessorius), and flexor digitorum brevis.[19] Clinically, the investigators tend to examine larger and more proximal muscles first, then progress distally and into smaller muscles. In this case, trigger point dry needling to the gastrocnemius may resolve both pain and range of motion complaints frequently seen with plantar fasciitis. For treatment of the lower limb pain, an acupuncturist may include needle placement in the thoracolumbar paraspinals to stimulate the sympathetic trunks to regulate neural connectivity and blood flow.

Concussion and whiplash injuries have become more common in dance choreography.[35] For example, a dancer may fall from a lift, be thrown into a set piece, or be kicked by another dancer. Although a typical concussion examination and neurologic assessment should always be performed, trigger points should also be assessed for their potential contribution to pain, range of motion restriction, muscle weakness, and other symptoms after head trauma or whiplash injury. The sternocleidomastoid

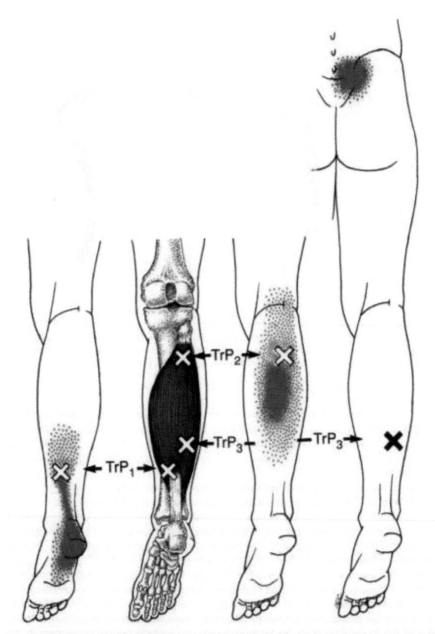

Fig. 3. Referral pattern from soleus to heel and arch of the foot. (*From* Donnelly JM, Fernande-de las-Penas C, Finnegan M, et al, eds. Travell, Simons & Simons' Myofascial Pain and Dysfunction. 3rd ed. Philadelphia, PA: Wolters Kluwer;2019:689; with permission.)

(SCM) muscle is often involved in concussion and whiplash injury due to the eccentric load that occurs with a coup-contrecoup mechanism.[36] Trigger points in the SCM may produce a variety of symptoms including, but not limited to, ipsilateral and contralateral headache, jaw pain, tinnitus and pressure in the ear, sinus pain, lacrimation,

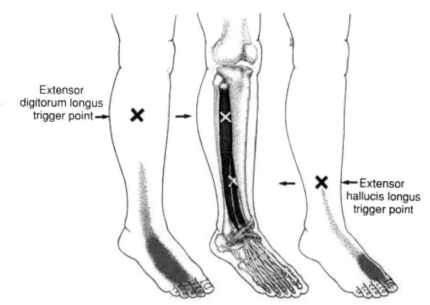

Extensor
digitorum longus
trigger point→

←Extensor
hallucis longus
trigger point

Fig. 4. Referral patterns from extensor digitorum longus and extensor hallucis longus. (*From* Donnelly JM, Fernande-de las-Penas C, Finnegan M, et al, eds. Travell, Simons & Simons' Myofascial Pain and Dysfunction. 3rd ed. Philadelphia, PA: Wolters Kluwer;2019:721; with permission.)

vertigo, etc.[36] Similarly, trigger points in the Longus colli and other deep cervical flexors may present as throat pain, a "lump" in the throat or difficulty swallowing, which are common symptoms after whiplash injury.[37] If the injury is chronic, insomnia and depression may affect the dancer's well-being and recovery potential. Acupuncture can help regulate the nervous system to reduce symptoms of depression[38] and insomnia.[39]

Dancers tend to have perfectionist tendencies and may present with higher levels of anxiety than their nondancer counterparts.[40] Clinically, this personality type may present with somatic manifestations, including frequent headaches and jaw pain.[41] Trigger points should be considered as contributing factors and the following muscles should be examined: suboccipitals, posterior cervical musculature, upper trapezius, levator scapulae, medial and lateral pterygoid, temporalis, masseter, and SCM.[18,31] This treatment approach also provides an opportunity to discuss other holistic care approaches, as the dancer may benefit from traditional acupuncture treatments to target anxiety and upregulation of the central nervous system.

Trigger points may also present as a result of acute injury. In an example of a dancer presenting with a lateral ankle sprain due to a plantar flexed and inverted landing, the fibularis longus, brevis, and tertius muscles may respond with trigger points due to eccentric overload sustained during the injury (**Fig. 5**). These trigger points may cause persistent lateral ankle pain. In addition, needling the fibular nerve may promote neuromuscular reeducation to improve impaired proprioception. A needle in the sinus tarsi (corresponding to traditional acupuncture point GB 40) is frequently used to treat ankle sprains. It likely interacts with local pain receptors and stimulates the injured tissue.[3]

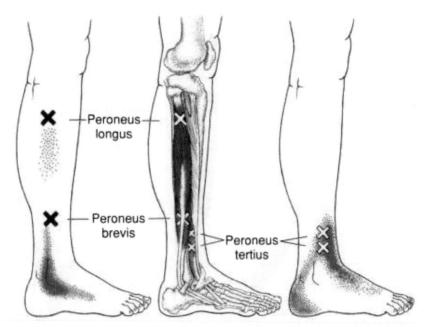

Fig. 5. Referral pattern from peroneus longus, brevis, and tertius muscles. (Fibularis longus, brevis, and tertius). (*From* Donnelly JM, Fernande-de las-Penas C, Finnegan M, et al, eds. Travell, Simons & Simons' Myofascial Pain and Dysfunction. 3rd ed. Philadelphia, PA: Wolters Kluwer;2019:581; with permission.)

TENDON, FASCIA, AND OTHER TISSUES

Although dry needling was initially used to treat trigger points, techniques are being reviewed to determine its efficacy in the treatment of tendinopathies, enthesopathies, fascial adhesions, and scar tissue. Significant improvement was demonstrated in lateral elbow pain with needle placement to 2 traditional acupuncture points (which are near the motor points of 2 of the muscles that insert via tendon to the lateral epicondyle).[42] This methodology demonstrates overlap of acupuncture and dry needling and how they may both be beneficial to the dancer. They are both systems that allow the practitioner to maximize the body's healing potential and resiliency as part of an adjunct to other manual therapies and neuromuscular reeducation. A variety of needle manipulation techniques are used, including rotations, pistoning, and fenestrations to achieve bleeding. More research in the management of tendinopathy is needed to examine the efficacy of needling techniques compared with traditional treatments (eccentric loading, cross-friction massage, fascial manipulation, ultrasound, laser therapy, etc.), and more invasive treatments (antiinflammatory injections, platelet rich plasma injections, stems cell injections, surgery, etc.). Clinically, these techniques may be particularly applicable to dancers presenting with patellar or Achilles tendinopathy. Because dancers suffer commonly from overuse tendinopathy pain, needling can be an important adjuvant to care.

TRAINING AND SCOPE OF PRACTICE

Both physicians and physical therapists can learn needling techniques to augment their treatment of dancers. The required qualifications for each practitioner vary among states and countries and will be governed by practice act statements. For example, physicians often receive trigger point injection training as part of their residency. They can obtain further training in either dry needling or acupuncture. Many requirements state that physicians complete a 300-hour acupuncture course before incorporating acupuncture within their practice. Dry needling is part of physical therapy (PT) practice as defined by the American Physical Therapy Association's statement in 2012.[13] However, at this time, physical therapists are not universally allowed to "puncture the skin," thus dry needling is not permitted in all areas. Where dry needling is permitted, some restrictions include requiring referral for dry needling from a physician, restricting the number of needles and specific procedures (such as being prohibited from electroacupuncture), number of years in practice before offering needling, number of training hours required, and specific tissues that can be treated. There has been litigation involving acupuncturists attempting to block physical therapists from performing dry needling, which has led to some inclusion of the PT practice acts that specifically differentiates dry needling from acupuncture techniques.[43] In addition, many dry needling training programs train practitioners in the differences between Western-based theories of dry needling and acupuncture techniques more related to Traditional Chinese Medicine. It is the responsibility of any health care practitioner to be familiar with practice statements from their professional organizations and the state in which they practice. In addition, physicians referring to PTs and other practitioners should be aware of statutes in their state.

Trigger points can also be effectively treated without the invasive intervention of dry needling. Sustained compression, with or without repeated contractions, may be used to treat most muscles in the body. Similarly, many acupuncture points may be treated manually with acupressure techniques. These may be options for practitioners who are not permitted or do not wish to use needling techniques. In addition, some patients are not appropriate for needling interventions, as discussed later.

SAFETY CONCERNS

Overall, acupuncture and dry needling are both extremely safe techniques when performed by practitioners with adequate training. A recent article examined 17 systematic reviews on safety of acupuncture. The conclusion states: "Minor and serious adverse events can occur during the use of acupuncture and related modalities, contrary to the common impression that acupuncture is harmless. Serious adverse events are rare, but need significant attention as mortality can be associated with them. Referrals should consider acupuncturists' training credibility, and patient safety should be a core part of acupuncture education."[44] In addition, a recent prospective study examining adverse events in dry needling treatments performed by physiotherapists in Ireland found that the upper risk rate for a significant adverse event is less than or equal to 0.04%.[45] Most of the serious adverse events that are reported in the literature were the result of penetration of the heart, lungs, or spinal cord, which is avoidable with care and proper precautions. Otherwise, minor adverse reactions such as ecchymosis and fatigue are transient and not usually limiting.[44,45]

There are muscles and patients in which dry needling may be a precaution or contraindication. For example, some training programs do not teach dry needling of the posterior tibialis muscle secondary to anatomic anomalies seen in the neurovascular structures in the deep posterior compartment. Some believe that needling this muscle may increase risk for bleeding and compartment syndromes. Other muscles may be more safely needled with use of ultrasound guidance.[46] Precaution should always be taken in needling patients on anticoagulant therapy or with clotting disorders.

Needling muscles in which direct hemostasis cannot be applied, that is, lateral ptery-goid and psoas major muscle belly, would be a contraindication due to an increased risk of bleeding. In the case of pregnancy, needling in the first trimester and in and around the abdominal wall, lumbar spine, and pelvis may be discouraged. Localized or systemic infection, metastasis, breast or pectoral implants, communication bar-riers, and fear of needles are other examples of cases in which manual treatment of trigger points may be recommended in lieu of dry needling.

In the case of a dancer, dry needling may be avoided 24 to 48 hours before perfor-mance due to the potential for residual soreness and alterations in muscle firing and patterning. This is determined on a case-by-case basis, and the patient's prior response to dry needling should always be considered. As with any intervention, acupuncture, dry needling, and trigger point treatment must always be used in conjunction with other manual therapies, therapeutic exercises, and neuromuscular reeducation as appropriate. With any needling therapy, there is potential for "too much of a good thing." Prolonged periods of exposure may induce excessive produc-tion of CCK-8 and deplete some of the substances that are likely to influence results.[47] Dry needling has been shown to be dose dependent, and excessively needling an area may increase tissue concentrations of substance P, tumor necrosis factors, among other nociceptive chemicals.[48]

SUMMARY

The role of the health care practitioner, whether physician, physical therapist, or acupuncturist, is to decrease pain and restore function in the short term and to restore adaptive potential and neural connectivity in the long term. When dysfunction is treated, pain improves. Acupuncture and dry needling improve tissue perfusion by improving vasomotor control and can improve strength by removing motor inhibition. Needling techniques can influence tissue healing, cell metabolism, tissue remodeling, and adhesions by improving tissue trophism. They work to decrease pain perception by influencing both nociceptive and central pain neuromodulators. Acupuncture and dry needling are safe, complementary modalities aimed at improving the function of the dancer.

CLINICS CARE POINTS

- Myofascial pain is common and should be included on the differential when eval-uating dancers.
- Trigger point pain referral patterns often mimic pain complaints and injuries that are frequently sustained by dancers.
- Acupuncture and dry needling are tools that can improve pain and function.
- Needling techniques are safe and effective when practiced by trained professionals.

DISCLOSURE

The authors have nothing to disclose.

REFERENCES

1. White A. Western medical acupuncture: a definition. Acupunct Med 2009; 27:33–5.
2. Li YM. Acupuncture journey to America: A turning point in 1971. J Tradit Chin Med 2015. https://doi.org/10.1016/j.jtcms.2015.03.001.

3. Claraco A. Contemporary Acupuncture for the Health Professionals. presentation presented at the: Contemporary Acupuncture for the Health Professionals Course; 2011; Hamilton, February 18, 2011.

4. Wang Q, Mao L. Diencephalon as a cardinal neural structure for mediating 2 Hz- but not 100 Hz-electroacupuncture analgesia. Behav Brain Res 1990;37:148–56.

5. Lee J, Jang K. Electroacupuncture inhibits inflammatory edema and hyperalgesia through regulation of cyclooxygenase synthesis in both peripheral and central nociceptive sites. Am J Chin Med 2006;34(6):981–8.

6. Reddy I, Dung H. Acupuncture: an anatomical approach. 2nd edition. Boca Raton (FL): Routledge; 2013.

7. Wen G, He X, Lu Y. Effect of acupuncture on neurotransmitters/modulators. In: Xia Y, Cao X, Wu G, et al, editors. Acupuncture therapy for neurological diseases. Berlin: Springer; 2010. p. 120–42.

8. Sobrian S, Walters E. Enhanced satellite cell activity in aging skeletal muscle after manual acupuncture-induced injury. Chin Med 2014;4(1):22–33.

9. Claraco A. Neurofunctional Acupuncture on the Treatment of Sports Injuries and the Protection of Athletic Performance: An Integrated Neuromechanical Model. presentation presented at the: Contemporary Acupuncture; May 3, 2012; Toronto.

10. Claraco A. Neurofunctional treatment of pain and dysfunction. Contemporary Medical Acupuncture Program. Presented at the Contemporary Acupuncture for the Health Professionals. Hamilton, February 18, 2011.

11. Napadow v, Kettner n, Liu J. Hypothalamus and amygdala response to acupuncture stimuli in carpal tunnel syndrome. Pain 2007;130:254–66.

12. Maeda y, kim h, kettner n. Rewiring the primary somatosensory cortex in carpal tunnel syndrome with acupuncture. Brain 2017;140:914–37.

13. American Physical Therapy Association. Physical Therapists & the Performance of Dry Needling: An Educational Resource Paper.; 2012.

14. Dorsher PT, Fleckenstein J. Trigger Points and Classical Acupuncture Points, Part 1: Qualitative and Quantitative Anatomic Correspondences. German Journal of Acupuncture and Related Techniques 2008;51(3):15–24.

15. Shah J, Gilliams E. Uncovering the biochemical milieu of myofascial trigger points using in vivo microdialysis: an application of muscle pain concepts to myofascial pain syndrome. J Bodyw Mov Ther 2008;12(4):371–84.

16. Lewit K. The needle effect in the relief of myofascial pain. Pain 1979;6:83–90.

17. Dommerholt J, Fernandez-de-las-Penas C. Trigger point dry needling. 2nd edition. Elsevier; 2018.

18. Simons D, Travell J, Simons L. 2nd edition. Travell and Simons' myofascial pain and dysfunction: the trigger point manual, vol. 1. Philadelphia: Williams & Wilkins; 1999.

19. Simons D, Travell J, Simons L. 2nd edition. Travell and Simons' myofascial pain and dysfunction: the trigger point manual, vol. 2. Philadelphia: Williams & Wilkins; 1999.

20. Gerwin RD, Dommerholt J, Shah J. An expansion of Simons' integrated hypothesis of trigger point formation. Curr Pain Headache Rep 2004;8(6):468–75.

21. Ga H, Koh H, Choi J, et al. Intramuscular and nerve root stimulation vs lidocaine injection to trigger points in myofascial pain syndrome. J Rehabil Med 2007; 39(5):374–8.

22. Hendler N, Kozikowski J. Overlooked physical diagnoses in chronic pain patients involved in litigation. Psychosomatics 1993;34:494–501.

23. Lucas K, Rich P, Polus B. Muscle activation patterns in the scapular positioning muscles during loaded scapular plane elevation: the effects of latent myofascial trigger points. Clin Biomech 2010;25(8):765–70.

24. Vecchiet L, Giamberardino M, Dragini L. Latent myofascial trigger points: changes in muscular and subcutaneous pain thresholds at trigger point and target level. J Manag Med 1990;5:151–4.

25. Bukhaveraeva E, Salakhutdinov R, Vyskocil F, et al. Spontaneous quantal and non-quantal release of acetylcholine at mouse endplate during onset of hypoxia. Physiol Res 2005;54:251–5.

26. Deval E, Gasull X, Noal J. Acid-sensing ion channels (ASICs): pharmacology and implications in pain. Pharmacol Ther 2010;128:549–58.

27. Ge H, Zhang Y, Boudreau S. Induction of muscle cramps by nociceptive stimulation of latent myofascial trigger points. Exp Brain Res 2008;187(4):623–9.

28. Hong C, Torigoe Y. Electrophysiological characteristics of localized twitch responses in responsive taut bands of rabbit skeletal muscle. J Musculoskelet Pain 1994;2:17–43.

29. Sueki DG, Cleland JA, Wainner RS. A regional interdependence model of musculoskeletal dysfunction: research, mechanisms, and clinical implications. J Man Manip Ther 2013;21(2):90–102.

30. Zerei, et al. Added Value of Gluteus Medius and Quadratus Lumborum Dry needling in Improving knee Pain an dFunction in Female Athletes with Patellofemoral Pain Syndrome: A randomized Clinical Trial. Arch Phys Med Rehabil 2020; 101:265–74.

31. Donnelly J, Fernandez-de-las-Penas C, Finnegan M, et al. Travell, simons, & simons' myofascial pain & dysfunction: the trigger point manual. 3rd edition. Philadelphia: Wolters Kluwer; 2019.

32. Goulart M, O'Malley MJ, Hodgkins CW. Foot and Ankle Fractures in Dancers. Clin Sports Med 2008;27(2):295–304.

33. Kadel NJ, Teitz CC, Kronmal RA. Stress fractures in ballet dancers. Am J Sports Med 1992;20(4):445–9.

34. Ahonen J. Biomechanics of the foot in dance: a literature review. J Dance Med Sci 2008;12(3):99–108.

35. McIntyre L, Leiderbach M. Concussion knowledge and behaviors in a sample of the dance community. J Dance Med Sci 2016;20(2):79–88.

36. Alsalaheen B, Johns K, Bean R, et al. Women and men use different strategies to stabilize the head in response to impulsive loads: implications for concussion injury risk. J Orthop Sports Phys Ther 2019;49(11):779–86.

37. Poorbaugh K, Brismée J-M, Phelps V, et al. Late whiplash syndrome: a clinical science approach to evidence-based diagnosis and management. Pain Pract 2008;8(1):65–89.

38. Wang z, et al, Wang x. Acupuncture treatment modulates the corticostriatal reward circuitry in major depressive disorder. J Psychiatr Res 2017;84:18–26.

39. Cao h, Pan. Acupuncture for treatment of insomnia: a systematic review of randomized controlled trials. J Altern Complement Med 2009;15(11):1171–86.

40. Eusanio J, Thompson P, Jagie SV. Perfectionism, Shame, and Self-concept in Dancers: A Mediation Analysis. J Dance Med Sci 2014;18(3):106–14.

41. Giannakopoulos N, Keller L, Rammelsberg P, et al. Anxiety and depression in patients with chronic temporomandibular pain and in controls. J Dent 2010;38(5): 369–76.

42. Gadau z, zhang hp, wang fc, et al. A multi-center international study of Acupuncture for lateral elbow pain - Results of a randomized controlled trial. Eur J Pain 2020. https://doi.org/10.1002/ejp.1574.

43. Illinois General Assembly. Illinois physical therapy act. 2017. Available at: http://www.ilga.gov/legislation/ilcs/ilcs3.asp?ActID=1319&ChapterID=24. Accessed May 5, 2020.

44. Chan M, Wu X, Wu J. Safety of acupuncture: overview of systematic reviews. Sci Rep 2017;7(1):3369.

45. Brady S, McEvoy J, Dommerholt J, et al. Adverse events following trigger point dry needling: a prospective survey of chartered physiotherapists. J Man Manip Ther 2014;22(3):134–40.

46. Shin H, Shin J. Application of Ultrasound-Guided Trigger Point Injection for Myofascial Trigger Points in the Subscapularis and Pectoralis Muscles to Post-Mastectomy Patients: A Pilot Study. Yonsei Med J 2014;55(3):792–9.

47. Han J, Ding X. Cholecystokinin octapeptide (CCK-8): Antagonism to electroacupuncture analgesia and a possible role in electroacupuncture tolerance. Pain 1986;27:101–15.

48. Hsieh Y, Yang S, Yang C, et al. Dry needling at myofascial trigger spots of rabbit skeletal muscles modulates the biochemicals associated with pain, inflammation, and hypoxia. Evid Based Complement Alternat Med 2012;2012:342165.

New Directions in Dance Medicine

Dancers with Disabilities, Blindness/Low Vision, and/or Deafness/Hard of Hearing

Mary Dubon, MD[a,b,c,]*, Rebecca Siegel, MD[b,c], Judith Smith[d],
Mark Tomasic, MFA[e], Merry Lynn Morris, MFA, PhD[f]

KEYWORDS

- Integrated dance • Inclusive dance • Dancers with disabilities • Adaptive dance
- Dance and disability • Dance medicine

KEY POINTS

- Dancers with disabilities, blindness/low vision, and/or deafness/hard of hearing (DWDBD) have received little attention in the dance medicine and science literature in terms of specific needs for healthy dance participation.
- Programs and companies for DWDBD continue to grow; thus, it is crucial that dance medicine begins to address the unique medical, injury prevention, and injury treatment considerations of DWDBD to facilitate their health and longevity in dance.
- The approach to safe and effective practices must be sufficiently nuanced in terms of both dance training and medical approach/treatment, because of the variety and uniqueness of DWDBD.
- Existing knowledge from dance medicine and para sports medicine can offer useful guidance, such as preparticipation physicals to support health, well-being, and injury prevention.
- More research is needed to better provide specific recommendations for DWDBD.

INTRODUCTION

Although dance medicine is a growing field, filled with up-to-date information on ways to promote healthy dance participation among recreational to elite dancers, to date, there has been little focus on dancers with disabilities, blindness/low vision, or

[a] Boston Children's Hospital, 300 Longwood Avenue, Boston, MA 02115, USA; [b] Spaulding Rehabilitation Hospital, 300 1st Avenue, Boston, MA 02129, USA; [c] Harvard Medical School, 25 Shattuck Street, Boston, MA 02115, USA; [d] AXIS Dance Company, 1428 Alice Street Suite 200, Oakland, CA 94612, USA; [e] Santa Monica College, 1900 Pico Boulevard, Santa Monica, CA 90405, USA; [f] University of South Florida, 4202 East. Fowler Avenue, Tampa, FL 33612, USA
* Corresponding author.
E-mail address: mary.dubon@childrens.harvard.edu

Phys Med Rehabil Clin N Am 32 (2021) 185–205
https://doi.org/10.1016/j.pmr.2020.09.010
1047-9651/21/© 2020 Elsevier Inc. All rights reserved.

pmr.theclinics.com

deafness/hard of hearing (DWDBD). For the purposes of this article, DWDBD refers to dancers with physical disabilities (affecting physical functioning, such as spinal cord injury or amputation), intellectual/developmental disabilities (IDDs; affecting intellectual functioning and adaptive behavior or developmental/social skills, such as Down syndrome, fragile X syndrome, or autism spectrum disorders), blindness/low vision, or deafness/hard of hearing. Other than anecdotal information, little is known about injury patterns, injury prevention, or wellness strategies for DWDBD. However, there are increasing numbers of dance programs and companies involving DWDBD at preprofessional and professional levels. Dance teachers and choreographers may now encounter a more diverse terrain when training dancing bodies, and this requires a significant reexamination of traditional practices. This article reviews the history and experience of DWDBD and explores dance medicine considerations relevant to working with DWDBD.

A BRIEF HISTORY OF INCLUSIVE/INTEGRATED DANCE

Although it is difficult to find a clear and comprehensive history of integrated, mixed-ability, or inclusive dance, efforts in this area of dance training and practice have been in development for many decades. This article highlights some important historical moments, acknowledging that this brief summation does not capture a thorough history. In 1955, Gallaudet University, a university for deaf/hard-of-hearing (DHH) students, founded Gallaudet Dance Company, a premier dance company that still continues.[1] In Vasteras, Sweden, in 1975, the first competition for para dance sport (then called wheelchair dance sport), which is adapted from ballroom dance and uses the rules of the World Dance Sports Federation applied for dancers with physical disabilities affecting their lower extremities, occurred. Para dance sport became officially governed by the International Paralympic Committee in 1998.[2] In the 1980s, physically integrated dance companies, such as AXIS Dance Company and Dancing Wheels, began with professional performance goals, focused on producing high-quality choreographic work involving individuals with and without disabilities.[3,4] Around this time, Alvin Ailey and Martha Graham began pioneering techniques to teach dance to blind students.[5] In 2002, Boston Ballet partnered with Boston Children's Hospital to create a dance class for dancers with Down syndrome.[6] Several similar programs have followed. In 2013, the International Bay Area Deaf Dance Festival was founded.[7] In 2017, Blind Dance Company was founded.[8] In 2019, dance sport was recognized as an official sport of Special Olympics International.[9] At the time of the writing of this article, many dance companies and dance programs exist for DWDBD; however, more work still needs to be done to provide recreational to elite opportunities for DWDBD.

Initially, DWDBD frequently learned movement skills through choreographic processes because there was an absence of training opportunities geared toward professional or preprofessional dance.[10] However, a variety of integrated dance companies now hold workshop intensives, teacher trainings, and community classes. Alito Alessi's DanceAbility International offered the first teacher training certification program for integrated/inclusive dance focusing on improvisation in 1996, and, in 2012, Dancing Wheels produced a teaching manual, focused on contemporary dance technique.[11,12] The International Bay Area Deaf Dancer Festival offers dance workshops for DHH dancers.[7] The Royal Ballet offers ballet classes geared toward blind/low-vision (BLV) dancers.[13] Boston Ballet offers dance teacher training for adaptive dance for dancers with Down syndrome and/or autism spectrum disorders.[14] However, more consistent, well-developed training opportunities in different locations are needed.[15]

The integrated/inclusive dance field is in a time of exceptional growth, making this article both relevant and timely. In July 2015, Dance/NYC held a conference entitled Dance. Disability. Artistry, a multiyear initiative coinciding with the 25th anniversary of the Americans with Disability Act.[16] A research report was compiled reporting on the conference discussions, outcomes, and recommendations for future efforts in dance and disability. Furthermore, in May 2016, the first National Convening on the Future of Physically Integrated Dance in the USA was held in New York.[17] As a continuation and outgrowth of the National Convening, 6 regional convening conferences discussing the future of the field were then held throughout the country. The convenings addressed challenges in the field, such as artistic quality, resources, training, recruitment, and sustainability.[17] Shortly after these conferences, Dance/USA, a United States national service organization dedicated to professional dance, created a Deaf and Disability Affinity Group.[18] Although knowledge of safe dance practices for DWDBD is scarce, there are efforts being made and it is hoped that this article can contribute to these efforts as well.

RATIONALE

To our knowledge, little literature exists on dance medicine considerations for DWDBD. Organizations such as International Association for Dance Medicine & Science, Performing Arts Medicine Association, and Dance/USA provide excellent guidance on how to keep dancers healthy through injury prevention, injury surveillance, appropriate nutrition, and mental health resources.[18–20] Many of these considerations for dancers in general have overlap for DWDBD; however, there may be key differences. This article offers guidance on the topic of dance medicine considerations for DWDBD based on the limited research and evidence that exists, extrapolation from para/adaptive sports medicine literature, and expert opinion. However, more research is needed in this important area of dance medicine.

THE DISABILITY SPECTRUM IN INTEGRATED/INCLUSIVE DANCE

As introduced earlier, various professional dance groups exist that are uniquely positioned for professional DWDBD. Some of these dance companies are specifically geared toward individuals with specific types of disabilities, whereas other groups are inclusive for dancers with various disabilities, and others are also inclusive for DWDBD and dancers without disabilities. **Table 1** reviews elite dance groups, including professional dance companies, dance competitions, and dance sport groups highlighting dancers with physical disabilities. Although there is not 1 centralized means of finding all professional dance companies geared toward inclusion of individuals with physical disabilities, AXIS Dance Company has information on their Web site about other physically integrated dance companies and organizations.[21]

Table 2 explores elite dance groups, including professional dance companies highlighting DHH and BLV dancers. Although the authors were unable to find specific elite dance companies, competition groups, or dance sport organizations geared toward professional dancers with IDD, there are many classes and programs specifically created with dancers with IDD in mind, as shown in **Table 3**.

It is important to acknowledge that not all DWDBD dance as part of a specific dance company, program, or competition group structured for DWDBD. Samantha Figgins, who is hard of hearing, is a professional dancer with Alvin Ailey American Dance Theater.[22] Philip Martin-Nelson is a professional dancer with autism who dances with Les Ballets Trockadero de Monte Carlo.[23] Mana Hashimoto is a blind choreographer who had sight until her 20s, so she has the unique experience of dancing with and without

Table 1
Professional dance companies, dance competition groups, or dance sport organizations that are physically integrated, physically inclusive, or specifically for dancers with physical disabilities

Dance Organization	Location	Web Site	Genre
Abilities Dance Boston	Boston, MA	https://www.abilitiesdanceboston.org	Contemporary/modern
Amici Dance Theatre Company	London, United Kingdom	https://amicidance.org	Dance theater
AXIS Dance Company	Oakland, CA	http://www.axisdance.org	Contemporary
Candoco	London, United Kingdom	https://candoco.co.uk	Contemporary/modern
Dancing Wheels	Cleveland, OH	https://dancingwheels.org	Contemporary/modern
DV8 Physical Theatre	London, United Kingdom	https://www.dv8.co.uk/projects	Contemporary/modern
Full Radius Dance	Atlanta, GA	https://ffullradiusdance.org	Contemporary/modern
Heidi Latsky Dance (The GIMP Project)	New York, NY	http://heidilatskydance.org	Contemporary/modern
Ill-Abilities	Montreal, CA	https://www.illabilities.com	Hip-hop
Infinite Flow: An Inclusive Dance Company	Sherman Oaks, CA	https://www.infiniteflowdance.org/home	Ballroom
Infinity Dance Theater	New York, NY	https://www.infinitydance.com/	Ballet and modern
Jess Curtis Gravity	San Francisco, CA	https://www.jesscurtisgravity.org/about-gravity	Contemporary/modern
Karen Peterson and Dancers	Miami, FL	https://www.karenpetersondancers.org/	Contemporary/modern
Kinetic Light	New York, NY	https://kineticlight.org/about	Contemporary/modern
Momenta	Chicago, IL	http://momentadances.org	Contemporary/modern
Remix Dance Company	Capetown, South Africa	https://www.myguidecapetown.com/things-to-do/remix-dance-company	Contemporary/modern
Restless Dance	Adelaide, South Australia	http://restlessdance.org	Contemporary/modern
REVolutions Dance	Tampa, FL	http://www.revdance.org/	Contemporary/modern
Rollettes	Los Angeles, CA	https://www.rollettesdance.com	Dance team
Stop Gap Dance Company	Farnham, United Kingdom	https://www.stopgapdance.com	Contemporary/modern
World Para Dance Sport	International	https://www.paralympic.org/dance-sport	Ballroom

Noncomprehensive list of national/international professional dance companies, dance competition groups, or dance sport organizations that either define themselves as a physically integrated dance company (employee dancers both with and without a physical disability) or companies in which all dancers have a physical disability.

Table 2
Dance professional dance companies highlighting deaf/hard-of-hearing and/or blind/low-vision dancers

Dance Companies Highlighting Deaf/Hard of Hearing Dancers	Location	Web Site	Genre
Company 360	Washington DC	https://www.companythreesixty.com	Contemporary/modern
Signdance Collective International	London, United Kingdom	https://www.signdancecollectiveinternational.com	Signdance theater
Urban Jazz Dance Company	San Francisco, CA	https://www.realurbanjazzdance.com/mr-antoine-hunter.html	Urban jazz dance
Gallaudet Dance Company	Washington DC	https://www.gallaudet.edu/department-of-art-communication-and-theatre/gallaudet-dance-company	Modern/tap/jazz/incorporation of american sign language
Taiwan First Deaf Dance Group	Taiwan	https://www.facebook.com/taiwanfirstdeafdance/	Contemporary/modern
Dance Companies Highlighting Blind/Low Vision Dancers			
Wild Zappers	United States	http://www.invisiblehands.com/wildzappers.html	Jazz/funk/hip-hop
The Blind Dance Company	Culver City, CA	https://theblinddanceco.org/?fbclid=IwAR3Z6-sFV58N9dkyckB3hRyQXSQrlot87gtnFijiuVuY_lBCfaSKbX6XwKBw	Latin/hip-hop/ballroom

Noncomprehensive list of national/international professional dance companies that either define themselves as an integrated dance company, employing dancers both with and without deafness/hard of hearing or blindness/low vision, or companies in which all company members are BLV or DHH dancers.

Table 3
Dance programs for dancers with intellectual/developmental disabilities

Dance Program	Location	Diagnosis	Web Site
Arts for Autism	Miami, FL	Autism spectrum	https://www.spectrumdancetherapy.com
Ballet for All Kids	Los Angeles, CA New York, NY	Autism spectrum, developmental disabilities, physical disabilities, sensory disability, ADHD	https://www.balletforallkids.com
Be Beautiful Be Yourself: Global Down Syndrome Foundation	Denver, CO	Down syndrome	https://www.globaldownsyndrome.org/programs-conferences-grants/programs/be-beautiful-be-yourself-dance-class-2/
Boston Ballet's Adaptive Dance Program	Boston, MA	Down syndrome Autism spectrum disorder	https://www.bostonballet.org/Home/Education/Program/All-ages-programming/Adaptive-Dance.aspx
Free 2 Be Me Dance	Los Angeles, CA Dublin, Ireland	Down syndrome	https://www.free2bemedance.org
New York City Ballet Workshops	New York, NY	Autism	https://www.nycballet.com/Educate/Access-Programs/Workshops-for-Children-with-Autism.aspx
Special Olympics Dance Sport	International	Intellectual disability	https://www.specialolympics.org/our-work/sports/dance-sport
United Dance	Amsterdam, New York, Paris, Boston, Burlington, Genval, Antwerp	Down syndrome	https://www.uniteddance.org/program

Noncomprehensive list of national and international programs that specialize in teaching dance to individuals with IDD.
Abbreviation: attention-deficit/hyperactivity disorder, attention-deficit/hyperactivity disorder.

sight.[24] In 2019, Sydney Mesher, a New York City Rockette with an upper extremity limb deficiency, became the Rockette's first known dancer with a visible disability.[25] Ali Stroker, Broadway's Oklahoma lead and Tony Award–winning actress, singer, and dancer, is a wheelchair user.[26,27]

ASSISTIVE DEVICES FOR USE IN DANCE

For a dancer with a physical disability, an assistive device (AD) can be integral to the dancer's experience. It is important to acknowledge that, similar to sport-specific devices, dance-specific ADs are typically not covered by insurance. There may be financial barriers to accessing ADs, particularly those that may be dance specific (such as a prosthetic device with a foot in the en pointe position). **Table 4** reviews grant organizations that may be helpful for individuals looking for assistance in supporting their dance-specific ADs. Many of these organizations provide assistance for athletic adaptive equipment through an application process.

Dance Wheelchairs

Depending on the physical disability, dancers may use manual wheelchairs, manual wheelchairs with power assist, or power wheelchairs for dancing. Manual wheelchairs for para dance sport often have 5 wheels, with 2 swivel casters anteriorly, 2 drive wheels, and 1 swivel caster posteriorly. A footplate is used to position and secure the dancer's feet and has the anterior swivel casters attached beneath it. This 5-wheeled setup allows smooth gliding transitions while maintaining stability to prevent tipping.[28] **Fig. 1**A shows a sample para dance sport wheelchair design.[2] In other dance forms, tipping is part of the movement strategy and this type of chair would

Table 4
Funding resources for assistive devices or adaptive equipment

	Funding Resource	Web Site
Nonspecific equipment for sports	Challenged Athletes Foundation	http://www.challengedathletes.org/programs/grants/
	Disabled Sports USA: grants	https://www.disabledsportsusa.org
	GoHawkeye Enabling Grant Program	https://gohawkeye.org/grants/
	High Fives nonprofit foundation	https://highfivesfoundation.org/
	IM Able Foundation	https://imablefoundation.org/programs/
	J-Rob Foundation	http://www.jrobfoundation.com/grant-application.html
	Kelly Bush Foundation: The Active Fund	https://kellybrushfoundation.org/
	PossAbilities	https://teampossabilities.org/grants-scholarships/
	Who Says I Can't	https://whosaysicant.org
Prosthetics for sports	Heather Abbot Foundation;	https://heatherabbottfoundation.org
	Jordan Thomas Foundation	https://jordanthomasfoundation.org
	Team Amputee Blade Runners	https://amputeebladerunners.com
	The Given Limb Foundation	https://givenlimb.org
	Wiggle Your Toes	https://www.wiggleyourtoes.org

A noncomprehensive list of different funding resources that can assist with funding for adaptive sports equipment.

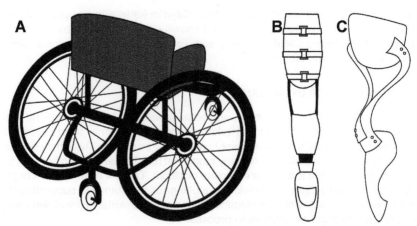

Fig. 1. Assistive device examples for dance. (*A*) A para dance sport wheelchair. (*B*) A prosthetic with a socket that allows for an interchangeable foot component, which in this case is a foot for pointe work (based on the prosthetic of Gabi Shull, social media influencer, dancer, amputee). (*C*) A dance-specific prosthetic, the Marie-T. ([*A-B*] *Courtesy of* R. Connaughton, PhD, Boston, MA. [*C*]*Courtesy of* R. Connaughton, PhD, Boston, MA and J. An, Seongnam-si, Korea.)

not be optimal. For instance, for a contemporary dancer who would like the ability to tip, this level of stability is not preferred, and, instead, a lightweight sports wheelchair without antitippers may be used. Sports wheelchairs should be lightweight, roll easily, and custom form fitting. The wheelchair seating system should have a snug fit, likened to the importance of a well-fitted shoe; have a stable base of support; and be optimized for prevention of pressure ulcers (eg, with a pressure-relieving cushion).[29,30] One strategy for determining whether the seating system is fitted properly is to have the wheelchair user do the twist. The wheelchair should move with the individual.[30] There should be at least 50 to 75 mm (2–3 inches) between the anterior edge of the seat and the popliteal angle to result in appropriate fit and seating positioning within the chair to set the dancer in an appropriate posture for optimal biomechanics with decreased risk of injury and pressure ulcers. The elbow angle when the hand is at the superior midportion of the push rim should be 90° to 120° for appropriate biomechanics of wheelchair propulsion. The seat height, seat dump (angle of the seat with respect to the horizontal plane of the chair), and wheel diameter all affect these angles and can be adjusted to allow the proper fit.[30]

Power wheelchair users may use their power wheelchairs to create smooth gliding movements of their chairs for dance. Some dancers have a manual wheelchair that has power-assist capability; for instance, a joystick power assist that may function in a similar fashion to a power wheelchair in terms of gliding movement ability. Separately, but perhaps of interest, Dr Merry Lynn Morris, in collaboration with engineers, designed a prototype power wheelchair that moves omnidirectionally and can be controlled hands free through leaning or tilting actions.[31,32]

Dance Prosthetics

Dancers with upper extremity amputations or limb deficiencies may choose to dance without the use of an upper extremity prosthetic or they may use a passive hand, padded hook, externally powered prosthetic hand, or an energy-storing Super Sport mitt (eg, for tumbling/acrobatics/handstands), depending on the desired functional use of the prosthetic.[33]

Dancers with lower extremity amputations or limb deficiencies also may choose to dance without the use of a prosthetic, though dancers often choose to dance with a prosthetic. When determining a dancer's prosthetic, it is important to have an understanding of the dance genre, dance-specific needs for the device, and functional needs for the prosthetic outside of dance. In some cases, a prosthetic may be able to be prescribed that can be used both for dance and for daily functional use. In some instances, a dance-specific prosthetic, separate from a functional day-to-day prosthetic, may be most beneficial for optimal dance performance. In other cases, the daily socket can be used both for day-to-day use as well as dance use, with interchangeable foot and/or knee components depending on the activity.[34,35]

Socket liners composed of elastomeric gel can be helpful to decrease shear stresses from the multidirectional forces that are often expected with athletic activities. Socket fit and comfort are important for athletic and artistic ability as well as for safety, because prosthetic sockets that are poorly fitted can result in skin breakdown, shear, or blistering. Shock-absorbing foot components should be considered and, in cases where additional shock absorption is required, shock-absorbing pylons can be placed between the socket and the prosthetic foot.[34]

In recent years, dance-specific prosthetics and dance-specific prosthetic components have gained media attention. Social media influencer and adolescent dancer Gabi Shull's story became known across the United States because she was a dancer before and after the diagnosis of osteosarcoma and subsequent Van Nes rotationplasty (surgery in which the tumor is resected and the tibia is rotated 180° and fixed to the femur so that the ankle joint acts like a knee joint) followed by return to dance with use of prosthetics.[36,37] Gabi has shared dance videos in which she performs tap or contemporary dance using 1 prosthetic foot and then is seen changing the foot component on her socket to a pointe-specific component to dance en pointe, similar to that seen in **Fig. 1B**.[36,38] Separately, the Marie-T prosthetic is an example of a dance-specific single-use (meaning for dance only) prosthetic that was designed to allow dancers with below-knee amputations to dance en pointe on their amputated legs (**Fig. 1C**).[39,40] This design features a three-dimensional–printed socket, carbon fiber brace, with rotational molded foot, stainless steel toe, and rubber grip toe.[40]

For dancers who choose not to use prosthetics on their upper or lower extremities, a custom limb protector may be beneficial, particularly in instances where the limb may be used for weight bearing.[34]

Other Dance Adaptive Devices and Braces

Dancers may have other ADs or braces that they wear in the community and/or that may be useful during dance. Crutches, walkers, canes, or braces used in the community may or may not be the optimal devices or braces for use in dance, as is the case for wheelchairs and prosthetics, as discussed earlier. For instance, Bill Shannon, known as the Crutch Master, uses shock-absorbing fuel hoses at the bottom of each crutch to provide an improved grip while mobilizing through space.[41] Similar to the design of the appropriate wheelchair or prosthetic, a good history of the type of dance and the desired use of the device is critical in determining an appropriate device. Working together with a creative rehabilitation team that may include the dancer (and, in some cases, the dance teacher or choreographer), a physiatrist, a prosthetist, an orthotist, a physical therapist, an occupational therapist, and/or vendor is key in the design of the appropriate, often customized, device.

DANCE CONSIDERATIONS FOR DANCERS WITH DISABILITIES, BLINDNESS/LOW VISION, AND DEAFNESS/HARD OF HEARING
Dance Considerations for Dancers with Physical Disabilities

Embodiment is an inroad to identity, to desire, to value formation, to body image, to competence, and to a sense of agency.[42,43] The uniquely embodied way the device is used in dance contrasts with the normative perception often associated with a medical aid. Medical aids are traditionally understood as utility-oriented devices designed to fulfill basic activities of daily living and serving a type of rehabilitative purpose. They often are associated with a negative stigma.[44,45] In dance, medical aids may be reimagined as creative catalysts facilitating an artistic intention, such as turning the device on its side or upside down to enable intriguing movement configurations and interactions, weight shifting off the vertical axis to evoke a flying or suspension quality, or using the device's shape or materiality to highlight a visual aesthetic or rhythmic dynamic. Although, traditionally, a cane is used to prevent falling, in dance, the dancer might use the cane to strategically fall in a way that reveals an expressive purpose or idea. In the dance context, what the AD is and how it is supposed to function may be radically upended. The wheelchair, crutch, or cane is transformed as a creative, embodied instrument outside the realm of traditional medical notions. For AD users in dance, the device often becomes an intimate part of the body, connected to the dancer's identity. This point is important, because it has implications for training and for how medical practitioners, teachers, and choreographers understand and engage with AD users. The same considerations of personal space and agency that are applied when touching or interacting with another person's body parts apply to interaction with a person's AD. When the dancer and the mobility device are viewed as both unique and integrated in terms of mobility, the approach to therapy, rehabilitation, AD prescription, conditioning, and dance training can be appropriately developed.

In current contemporary physically integrated dance, professional dancers who use wheelchairs may be seen pitching the chair off axis; descending to the floor in the chair via rolling, sliding, tipping, hoisting, or combinations thereof; rolling in succession on the floor with the device; altering their bodily orientation in the device; spinning at high speeds; and adopting strategies for moving in and out of their chairs. Dancers who use wheelchairs may also perform complex partnering work that can involve lifting or carrying the weight of other dancers on their backs, shoulders, legs, and/or parts of their chairs. Techniques for counterbalancing in duet and group choreographic work are often used. All of these types of movements require careful coordination, strength, and control, which require specialized conditioning approaches and attention to bodily uniqueness. A research study of 8 professional dancers who use ADs (manual wheelchair [6]; crutch [1]; power wheelchair [1]) indicated that speed regulation, nuanced control, stability, ideal seat positioning for maneuverability and partnering, appropriate friction between device and flooring, and a lightweight, small frame were high priorities for dancers who use ADs.[46]

Again, not all dancers with physical disabilities use ADs. For dancers with physical disabilities who do not use ADs, physical accommodations may still be necessary, as in the examples of an individual with asymmetry from a unilateral amputation or a neurologic condition affecting coordination. Dance instructors/choreographers should work with each dancer on the individual accommodations and the individual movement interpretation.

Dance Considerations for Dancers with Intellectual/Developmental Disabilities

Strategies should also be considered for dancers with IDDs. Consistent structured schedules/routines and clear visual aids for dance education can be beneficial for dancers with IDDs. For example, the Boston Ballet's ballet program for dancers with Down syndrome uses different colored tape on the right and left shoes for ease of following the directions of the dance teacher.[6] The dance teacher/choreographer should become aware of any sensory sensitivities the dancer has when considering props, footwear (or lack thereof), and costuming.[47]

Dance Considerations for Blind/Low-Vision Dancers

BLV dancers may require tactile cues and clear verbal instructions to describe dance maneuvers and choreography, whereas dance teachers/choreographers have traditionally been trained to depend more heavily on visual cues.[5] Dancers may need to rely on their proprioceptive skills, strength, and, if applicable, tactile cues of dance partners.[5] Tactile modeling, during which the BLV dancer touches a model who is demonstrating a dance maneuver, can be a valuable tool used when teaching dance/choreography. An example is when Martha Graham was teaching Hellen Keller to jump and she asked what Martha Graham meant by this. Martha Graham had Hellen Keller place her hands on Merce Cunningham's back as Merce Cunningham demonstrated a jump.[5] Teaching dance or choreography typically involves an element of physical demonstration of the maneuvers. This method likely is adjusted when teaching BLV dancers, either with demonstrations in closer proximity or with guiding the dancer's body through tactile cues.[5]

Dance Considerations for Deaf/Hard-of-Hearing Dancers

DHH dancers may use vibrations or visual cues for learning dance/choreography. Clapping, which offers a visual component for keeping the beat, may be valuable.[48] Feel the Beat Dance Studio uses a unique technology to create a vibrational dance floor that optimizes DHH dancers' ability to feel the rhythm of the music.[49]

DANCE TEACHER/CHOREOGRAPHER CONSIDERATIONS

Dancer teachers with or without disabilities, blindness/low vision, or deafness/hard of hearing cannot assume their bodily experiences can easily approximate the bodily experiences of the individual DWDBD with whom they are working. Even among DWDBD, neurologic movement patterns and sensations can vary extensively. It is helpful for dance teachers and choreographers to be flexible and adapt to each individual and observe the dancer's pattern of movements or interpretations of movement, to try to put themselves in the position of the dancer (eg, for teachers or choreographers who do not use an AD, it may be beneficial to experiment in/with a similar AD when creating movement). DWDBD deserve the same right to be challenged, to fail, and to succeed as their counterparts. Movement vocabulary should be modified as skill levels increase to ensure physical, cognitive, and artistic development.

In designing movement vocabulary, instructors should be cognizant that adult students with disabilities may not have had access to early dance training. This lack of early training is caused by several factors, including a paucity of qualified instructors and relevant dance curricula as well as accessibility issues. In addition, because the prevalence of disabilities increases with age, many DWDBD come to the profession later in life.[50] DWDBD who are new to dance as adults are often placed in intermediate/advanced classes and pressured to catch-up with more experienced dancers.

Dance instructors, choreographers, and dance medicine physicians should be attentive to previous dance training, age of participants, and level of experience, and adjust exercises and expectations accordingly.

IMPLICATIONS FOR DANCE MEDICINE PRACTICE

Dance medicine physicians are trained and experienced in caring for the medical needs of dancers. Little has been known or addressed specifically to DWDBD. Although there are many overlapping areas, there are also many unique considerations for this population.

Preparticipation physicals are a mainstay for sports participation for youth and young adults in the United States; however, they are not a mainstay for dance participation. The authors strongly recommend dance-specific preparticipation physicals for health, well-being, and prevention of injury of all dancers, including DWDBD and dancers without disabilities, blindness/low vision, or deafness/hard of hearing. Interestingly, collegiate dancers have been shown to be not very likely to seek medical attention, particularly of a physician, for injuries.[51] Collegiate sports athletes typically have had preparticipation physicals performed throughout their youth sports careers leading up to and including college, but this is less likely to be the case for collegiate dancers, because it is not a universal requirement for dance participation throughout youth. There is concern that collegiate dancers may not seek the attention of a physician for injuries, which can potentially lead to progression of injury. Perhaps, if the dance culture also promoted screening by a health team for safety, injury education, and injury prevention, dancers would be more likely to seek medical help when concerns do arise.

The Dance/USA Task Force on Dancer Health has an extensive preseason posthire health screen for professional dancers that is composed of a health history questionnaire and a physical assessment performed by trained dance medicine clinicians (physical therapists, athletic trainers, and/or physicians). This preparticipation assessment is an excellent means of screening professional dancers for safe dance participation, while also screening for possible injury susceptibilities and means of decreasing these risks, allowing the dancers to best prepare for a healthy season. Dance/USA now has adaptations to its health screen for professional dancers with disabilities; for instance, substituting some lower extremity screening components for ambulatory dancers with upper extremity screening components for wheelchair users.[18]

Preparticipation physicals performed for sports often have supplemental considerations for athletes with disabilities.[52-54] Given the growing number of DWDBD, it is crucial that dance medicine begins to address the unique medical, injury prevention, and injury treatment considerations of DWDBD. **Table 5** reviews components of preparticipation examinations included in sports preparticipation history and physical examinations for athletes with disabilities.[52-54] The authors believe that these same considerations and principles should be applied to preparticipation physicals and health screens for recreational through elite DWDBD. The purpose of this is not discrimination but for inclusion and assurance that DWDBD are kept safe and healthy for long careers in their art form. It may be important, for instance, that precautions are known to allow safe dance participation. **Table 6** reviews common precautions/safety/medical considerations that should be considered for individuals based on diagnosis.[55-60]

Although there is a growing body of literature on injury patterns in athletes with disabilities, there is a lack of literature on injury patterns in DWDBD. For dancers with

Table 5
Components of preparticipation physical examinations for athletes with disabilities, deafness/hard of hearing, blindness/low vision

General PPE History Components	Recommended Additional PPE History Components for Athletes with Disabilities	PPE Components
Medical History:	AD use	Vitals
Allergies	Atlantoaxial instability	Constitutional/general
Anemia	Autonomic dysreflexia history or risk	Ear/eyes/nose/throat
Cardiac symptoms/conditions	Bladder function (including neurogenic bladder/need for catheterization and any related complications such as urinary tract infections)	Lymph nodes
Concussions/head injuries	Bowel function (including neurogenic bowel/need for a bowel program)	Cardiovascular
Diabetes	Classification for para sport (if known)	Respiratory
Dislocations	Dietary considerations, such as use of a gastrostomy tube	Abdominal
Eating disorders/disordered eating/weight concerns	Disability diagnosis/cause of disability (eg, spina bifida, amputation, CP, SCI)	Integumentary
Fainting (particularly with exercise)	Functional level of independence for mobility and other relevant activities of daily living	Neurologic
Fractures	Hearing loss/deafness	Musculoskeletal
Headaches with exercise	Hematologic condition/history of easy bleeding	—
Heat illness	Hepatitis	—
Hernias	Latex allergy	—
Hospitalizations	Low bone mineral density	—
Immunizations	Motor impairments	—
Infections (including mononucleosis, herpes, MRSA, or blood-borne pathogens such as HIV or hepatitis B or C)	Neurologic/functional changes in recent history	—
Medical conditions	Orthotic use	—
Medications	Other medical conditions or comorbidities	—
Menstrual history	Precautions/restrictions for exercise	—
Mental health screen	Prosthetic use	—
Missing organs	Renal disease/unilateral kidney	—
Muscle cramps caused by exercise	Sensory impairments	—

(continued on next page)

Table 5 (continued)		
General PPE History Components	**Recommended Additional PPE History Components for Athletes with Disabilities**	**PPE Components**
Neurologic symptoms/history	Skin breakdown/pressure ulcers	—
Other concerns to be discussed with clinician	Spasticity/dystonia	—
Respiratory conditions/ symptoms	Splenomegaly	—
Seizures	Thermoregulatory impairment	—
Sickle cell disease/trait	Visual loss/blindness	—
Skin concerns	—	—
Soft tissue injuries	—	—
Surgeries	—	—
Swollen joints	—	—
Vision history	—	—
Family history:	—	—
Cardiac conditions	—	—
Sickle cell disease/trait	—	—
Sudden/young death	—	—

This table, with some adjustments, summarizes recommendations for history and physical components for the PPE traditionally performed before sports activities. Most of the suggestions are from Ref.[54] with additional suggestions from Refs.52,53 and author expert opinion.

Abbreviations: CP, cerebral palsy; HIV, human immunodeficiency virus; MRSA, methicillin-resistant *Staphylococcus aureus*; SCI, spinal cord injury; PPE, preparticipation physical examination.

Adapted from Dubon ME, Rovito C, Van Zandt DK, Blauwet CA. Youth Para and Adaptive Sports Medicine. Curr Phys Med Rehabil Reports. 2019;7(2):104-115; with permission.

physical disabilities, extrapolation from adaptive sports medicine literature may be helpful until further literature is available for DWDBD. A critical review of the para sport literature revealed that athletes who were wheelchair users had a tendency toward upper extremity injuries (including shoulder, elbow, wrist, and hand injuries; muscle/tendon injuries; as well as mononeuropathies), whereas ambulatory athletes had a tendency toward lower extremity injuries.[61] Shoulder pain and injury are common in wheelchair users; however, research has shown that the odds of shoulder pain in nonathlete wheelchair users is greater than in wheelchair athletes, suggesting that strengthening and conditioning likely decreases the risk of shoulder pain.[62] The authors suspect that proper wheelchair propulsion biomechanics and periscapular strengthening are important for the shoulder health of wheelchair dancers; however, further research is needed to test this hypothesis.

Few data exist for injury patterns among dancers or any athletes with IDD. Limited data from Special Olympics indicate that musculoskeletal and skin concerns are frequent reasons for medical consultation at their large events; however, more research is needed on overall injury patterns among athletes and/or dancers with IDD.[63] Similarly, few data exist for BLV or DHH athletes or dancers. Football five-a-side is a Paralympic sport for BLV athletes. Research has shown a predominance of lower extremity, head, and neck injuries in this sport.[64] Given the significant

Table 6
Precautions/medical/safety considerations for athletes and dancers with disabilities, deafness/hard of hearing, and blindness/low vision

Condition	Precautions/Medical Considerations
Spinal cord injury	• Motor impairments • Sensory impairments • Pressure sores • Low bone mineral density • Spasticity • Neurogenic bladder • Neurogenic bowel • Thermoregulation impairments • At risk for autonomic dysreflexia
Cerebral palsy	• Motor impairments • Spasticity • Dystonia • Low bone mineral density • At risk for pressure ulcers • Orthopedic comorbidities • At risk for seizures
Spina bifida	• Motor impairments • Sensory impairments • At risk for pressure ulcers • Low bone mineral density • Hydrocephalus/shunt • Chiari malformation • Neurogenic bladder • Neurogenic bowel • Cognitive impairment • Tethered cord • Orthopedic comorbidities
Congenital limb deficiency/amputation	• At risk for pressure ulcers/blisters • Phantom limb sensation/pain • Risk of appositional bone growth/terminal overgrowth in youth
Muscular dystrophies	• Exercise restrictions: concern for muscle damage, particularly with eccentric exercise • Pulmonary comorbidities • Cardiac comorbidities • Low bone mineral density • At risk for pressure ulcers
Arthrogryposis	• Decreased range of motion • Motor impairments • Pressure sores
Postpoliomyelitis/acute flaccid myelitis	• Motor impairment • Low bone mineral density • Respiratory impairments • Cranial nerve impairments
Brain injury	• Motor impairments • Cognitive impairments • Coordination impairments • Vision difficulties • Hearing difficulties • Spasticity

(continued on next page)

Table 6 *(continued)*	
Condition	**Precautions/Medical Considerations**
	• Dystonia • Movement disorders • At risk for seizures • Sports clearance by physician needed after brain injury • Possible ongoing restrictions from contact/collision sports
IDDs	• Many types • Medical comorbidity with known diagnoses • Complications associated with medication side effects • Considerations for Down syndrome • Atlantoaxial instability • Cardiac comorbidities • Ligamentous laxity
Achondroplasia	• Foramen magnum narrowing increasing risk for cervical myelopathy • Hydrocephalus • Avoidance of gymnastics/tumbling/contact sports
Multiple sclerosis	• Motor impairments • Cognitive impairments • Spasticity • Sensory impairments • Neurogenic bladder • Neurogenic bowel • Optic neuritis • Low bone mineral density • At risk for pressure ulcers
Deafness/hard of hearing	• Associated renal disease • Associated balance difficulty • Associated visual impairment
Blindness/low vision	• Cause of visual impairment and associated comorbidity

Data from Refs.[55–60] Please refer to Ref.[55] for more details and more resources for a more in-depth review of the topic.

difference between this sport and dance, it is unclear whether these injury patterns are applicable for BLV dancers.

Disordered eating, female athlete triad (FAT)/relative energy deficiency in sport (RED-S), substance misuse, and mental health concerns associated with perfectionism have been reported in dancers; however, to our knowledge this has not been examined in DWDBD.[65–67] However, a recent study indicates that para athletes have factors traditionally associated with FAT/RED-S, highlighting the need for more research in this area for para athletes and DWDBD.[68]

When working with DWDBD, the general principles of dance medicine injury prevention should be applied, including the importance of dynamic stretching, conditioning, nutrition, and mental health support, but more research is needed in the area of injury patterns, injury prevention, and wellness in DWDBD to better provide more specific recommendations for this population.[69]

SUMMARY

Dance medicine is a growing field. Similarly, there is a growing number of dancers with disabilities, blindness/low vision, and deafness/hard of hearing. This article provides an overview of dance and dance medicine for individuals with disabilities, blindness/ low vision, and deafness/hard of hearing. Considerations for dancers with physical disabilities may include prescription of an appropriate AD and adjustments to physical movement with or without AD use. Dance considerations for BLV dancers may include use of tactile modeling, whereas considerations for DHH dancers may include use of visual cues or vibration of the floor. Dance considerations for dancers with IDDs may include use of memory strategies and visual aids to assist with remembering choreography and use of consistent structured class schedules. Little is known about dance injury patterns or wellness considerations for dancers with disabilities, low vision, or deafness/hard of hearing; however, the authors call for more research in this area and in the meantime recommend applying knowledge from dance medicine and para sports medicine. A high degree of collaboration and communication is vitally important for both dance professionals and health professionals working with DWDBD.

ACKNOWLEDGMENTS

The authors would like to acknowledge Cheri Blauwet, MD; Kristen Stevens; and Marijeanne Liederbach PhD, PT, ATC, CSCS, for their assistance with the content and creative process of this article.

DISCLOSURE

M. Dubon has received funding from National Curriculum Initiative in Developmental Medicine, Deborah Munroe Noonan Memorial Fund/Health Resources in Action, Med-Strat (spouse's stock, spouse employment), Amazon (spouse's stock)and is Special Olympics Massachusetts MedFest Medical Director and Special Olympics Consultant for Sports Prevention of Risk through Incident Tracking (SPRINT). R. Siegel, J. Smith, M. Tomasic and M.L. Morris have nothing to disclosure.

REFERENCES

1. Gallaudet dance company – Gallaudet university. Available at: https://www. gallaudet.edu/office-of-development/gallaudet-dance-company. Accessed May 9, 2020.
2. Para dance sport - about the sport | international Paralympic committee. Available at: https://www.paralympic.org/dance-sport/about. Accessed May 9, 2020.
3. About dancing wheels – dancing wheels. Available at: https://dancingwheels.org/ about-dancing-wheels-copy/. Accessed May 9, 2020.
4. Mission — AXIS dance company. Available at: https://www.axisdance.org/ mission. Accessed May 9, 2020.
5. Seham J, Yeo AJ. Extending our vision: access to inclusive dance education for people with visual impairment. J Dance Educ 2015;15(3):91–9.
6. Boston children's hospital. Adaptive dance - YouTube. Available at: https://www. youtube.com/watch?v=OkWlpYK77SA. Accessed May 9, 2020.
7. Bay area international deaf dance festival. Available at: https://www. realurbanjazzdance.com/bay-area-international-deaf-dance-festival.html. Accessed May 9, 2020.
8. Campodonico C. Moving blind: visually impaired performers dance from the soul - at this stage. Available at: https://thisstage.la/2017/08/moving-blind-visually-impaired-performers-dance-from-the-soul/. Accessed May 9, 2020.

9. Competitive cheer and dancesport adopted as recognized sports of special olympics. Available at: https://www.specialolympics.org/about/press-releases/competitive-cheer-and-dancesport-adopted-as-recognized-sports-of-special-olympics. Accessed May 9, 2020.

10. McGrath E. Dancing with disability: an intersubjective approach. In: Goodley Dan, Hughes Bill, Davis L, editors. Disability and social theory. Palgrave Macmillan UK; 2012. p. 143–58. https://doi.org/10.1057/9781137023001_9.

11. DanceAbility International I About Us. Available at: https://www.danceability.com/about-us. Accessed May 9, 2020.

12. Tomasic M, Verdi-Fletcher M. Dancing wheels (Dance group). Physically integrated dance training : the dancing wheels comprehensive guide for teachers, choreographers and students of mixed abilities. Cleveland (OH): NewVoices; 2012.

13. Schrock M. Go inside a dance class for the blind at the royal ballet - dance magazine 2017. Available at: https://www.dancemagazine.com/go-inside-dance-class-blind-royal-ballet-2307053887.html. Accessed May 9, 2020.

14. Boston ballet - education | adaptive dance teacher training. Available at: https://www.bostonballet.org/Home/Education/Resources/For-Educators/Adaptive-Dance-Training. Accessed May 9, 2020.

15. Aujla IJ, Redding E. The identification and development of talented young dancers with disabilities. Res Dance Educ 2014;15(1):54–70.

16. Disability. Dance. Artistry. | Dance/NYC. Available at: https://www.dance.nyc/programs/dancenyc-events/2015/07/Disability.-Dance.-Artistry/. Accessed May 9, 2020.

17. The Future of Physically Integrated Dance in the USA; 2017. Available at: https://static1.squarespace.com/static/53a9f1fbe4b08edefaf5367d/t/59a4840e6f4ca33 13b05c3fe/1503953949140/AxisDance-Report-DanceUSA2017-Final-AltTags%28lo-res%29.pdf.

18. Dance/USA — the national service organization for professional dance. Available at: https://www.danceusa.org/. Accessed May 9, 2020.

19. International association for dance medicine & science. Available at: https://www.iadms.org/. Accessed May 9, 2020.

20. Performing arts medicine association | dedicated to the health of performing artists. Available at: http://www.artsmed.org/. Accessed May 9, 2020.

21. Resources — AXIS dance company. Available at: https://www.axisdance.org/resources. Accessed May 9, 2020.

22. How Ailey's samantha figgins dances with hearing loss - dance spirit. Available at: https://www.dancespirit.com/samantha-figgins-single-sided-deafness-2635360817.html. Accessed May 9, 2020.

23. Making dance/movement therapy the therapy of choice for autism spectrum disorder | ADTA. Available at: https://adta.org/2015/04/20/making-dancemovement-therapy-the-therapy-of-choice-for-autism-spectrum-disorder/. Accessed May 9, 2020.

24. Greene M. What it's like to be a dancer & choreographer when you're blind. Dance magazine. 2018. Available at: https://www.dancemagazine.com/blind-dance-2621901530.html?rebelltitem=4#rebelltitem4. Accessed May 9, 2020.

25. del Valle L. First visibly disabled radio city rockette takes the stage - CNN. CNN. 2019. Available at: https://www.cnn.com/2019/12/24/us/disabled-radio-city-rockette-history-trnd/index.html. Accessed May 9, 2020.

26. Perron W. Ali Stroker: first wheelchair performer on Broadway - dance magazine. dance magazine. Available at: https://www.dancemagazine.com/ali-stroker-first-wheelchair-performer-on-broadway-2306985638.html. Accessed May 9, 2020.

27. Kim S. Ali Stroker's tony award was only Broadway's first step to disability inclusivity. Forbes. 2019. Available at: https://www.forbes.com/sites/sarahkim/2019/06/13/ali-stroker-tony-award/#cd410c17a734. Accessed May 9, 2020.

28. Caldwell M, De Luigi AJ. Wheelchair dance sport. In: De Luigi AJ, editor. Adaptive sports medicine. 1st edition. Springer International Publishing; 2018. p. 171–9. https://doi.org/10.1007/978-3-319-56568-2_16.

29. Cooper RA, De Luigi AJ. Adaptive sports technology and biomechanics: wheelchairs. PM R 2014;6(8 SUPPL). https://doi.org/10.1016/j.pmrj.2014.05.020.

30. Cooper RA, Cooper R, Susmarski A. Wheelchair sports technology and biomechanics. In: De Luigi AJ, editor. Adaptive sports medicine. 1st edition. Springer International Publishing; 2018. p. 21–34. https://doi.org/10.1007/978-3-319-56568-2_2.

31. Morris M, M R, Messerschmidt T, T L, Edmonston N. US patent for omni-directional remote-controlled mobility apparatus patent (Patent # 9,027,678 issued May 12, 2015) - Justia patents search. US Patient. 2015. Available at: https://patents.justia.com/patent/9027678. Accessed May 9, 2020.

32. Morris ML. Mobilizing possibilities: dance, disability and technology. J Humanit Rehabil . 2015. Available at: http://artsanddisability.blogspot.com. Accessed May 9, 2020.

33. Radocy B. Special considerations: upper-limb prosthetic adaptations for sports and recreation | o&p virtual library. atlas of limb prosthetics: surgical, prosthetic, and rehabilitation principles. Available at: http://www.oandplibrary.org/alp/chap12-03.asp. Accessed May 9, 2020.

34. De Luigi AJ. Technology and biomechanics of adaptive sports prostheses. In: De Luigi AJ, editor. Adaptive sports medicine. 1st edition. Springer International Publishing; 2018. p. 35–47. https://doi.org/10.1007/978-3-319-56568-2_3.

35. De Luigi AJ, Cooper RA. Adaptive sports technology and biomechanics: Prosthetics. PM R 2014;6(8 SUPPL). https://doi.org/10.1016/j.pmrj.2014.06.011.

36. Heigl A. Gabi shull: teen dancer uses prosthesis post-cancer | PEOPLE.com. People. 2016. Available at: https://people.com/celebrity/gabi-shull-teen-dancer-uses-prosthesis-post-cancer/. Accessed May 9, 2020.

37. Van Nes CP. Rotation-Plasty For Congenital Defects Of The Femur. J Bone Joint Surg Br 1950;32-B(1):12–6.

38. Zidepa L. This amputee defied the odds to become a ballerina | News24. You. 2016. Available at: https://m.news24.com/You/Archive/this-amputee-defied-the-odds-to-become-a-ballerina-20170728. Accessed May 9, 2020.

39. Marie . T — Jae-Hyun an. design. Available at: http://www.jaehyunan.com/new-page-45/. Accessed May 9, 2020.

40. Stahl J. There's a new prosthesis designed for dancing on pointe. Dance magazine 2018. Available at: https://www.dancemagazine.com/prosthetic-pointe-2618740374.html. Accessed May 9, 2020.

41. Davies T. Mobility: AXIS dancers push the boundaries of access. Text Perform Q 2008;28(1–2):8–42.

42. Standal ØF. Re-embodiment: incorporation through embodied learning of wheelchair skills. Med Health Care Philos 2011;14(2):177–84.

43. Iwakuma M. The body as embodiment: an investigation of the body by Merleau-Ponty. In: Corker M, Shakespeare T, editors. Disability, postmodernity, embodying disability theory. London (United Kingdom): Continuum; 2002. p. 76–87.

44. Jutai J, Day H. Psychosocial impact of assistive devices scale (PIADS). Technol Disabil 2002;14(3):107–11.

45. Scherer MJ, Sax C, Vanbiervliet A, et al. Predictors of assistive technology use: the importance of personal and psychosocial factors. Disabil Rehabil 2005; 27(21):1321–31.

46. Morris ML. Dance, disability, and assistive technology: probing interdisciplinary landscapes and re-imagining design 2017.

47. Cone TP, Cone SL. Strategies for Teaching Dancers of All Abilities. J Phys Educ Recreat Dance 2011;82(2):24–31. https://doi.org/10.1080/07303084.2011. 10598578.

48. Edelstein C. The link between american deaf culture and dance: assessing nonverbal communication and recognizing the value of deaf dancers 2016. Available at: https://digitalcommons.butler.edu/ugtheses. Accessed May 9, 2020.

49. How? — feel the beat dance. Available at: https://feelthebeat.dance/the-technology. Accessed May 9, 2020.

50. Brault M. Disability status and the characteristics of people in group quarters: a brief analysis of disability prevalence among the civilian noninstitutionalized and total populations in the American community survey 2008. Available at: http://www.census.gov/acs/www/Downloads/2006/usedata/Subject_Definitions.pdf. Accessed May 9, 2020.

51. Air ME, Grierson MJ, Davenport KL, et al. Dissecting the doctor-dancer relationship: health care decision making among American collegiate dancers. PM R 2014;6(3):241–9.

52. Dec KL, Sparrow KJ, McKeag DB. The physically-challenged athlete: medical issues and assessment. Sports Med 2000;29(4):245–58.

53. Siow HM, Cameron DB, Ganley TJ. Preparticipation sports evaluation: issues for healthy children and athletes with disabilities. J Pediatr Orthop 2010;30(SUPPL. 2):S17–20.

54. Bernhardt DT, Roberts WO. American academy of family physicians. PPE: preparticipation physical evaluation. 5th edition. Itasca: American Academy of Pediatrics; 2019.

55. Dubon ME, Rovito C, Van Zandt DK, et al. Youth para and adaptive sports medicine. Curr Phys Med Rehabil Rep 2019;7(2):104–15.

56. Palmer T, Weber KM. The deaf athlete. Curr Sports Med Rep 2006;5(6):323–6.

57. Official website of IBSA - international blind sports federation. Available at: http://www.ibsasport.org/. Accessed May 10, 2020.

58. Visually impaired friendly athletics a guide for supporting visually impaired adults and children in athletics. Available at: https://britishblindsport.org.uk/wp-content/uploads/2017/07/VisuallyImpairedFriendlyAthletics.pdf. Accessed May 10, 2020.

59. Court H, McLean G, Guthrie B, et al. Visual impairment is associated with physical and mental comorbidities in older adults: a cross-sectional study. BMC Med 2014;12(1):181.

60. Chandan P, Dubon ME. Clinical considerations and resources for youth athletes with intellectual disability: a review with a focus on special olympics international. Curr Phys Med Rehabil Rep 2019;7(2):116–25.

61. Tuakli-Wosornu YA, Mashkovskiy E, Ottesen T, et al. Acute and chronic musculoskeletal injury in para sport: a critical review. Phys Med Rehabil Clin N Am 2018; 29(2):205–43.

62. Fullerton HD, Borckardt JJ, Alfano AP. Shoulder pain: a comparison of wheelchair athletes and nonathletic wheelchair users. Med Sci Sports Exerc 2003;35(12): 1958–61.

63. Wheeler PC, Williamson T, Stephens C, et al. A report of the medical team activity at the 2009 Special Olympics GB. Br J Sports Med 2012;46(2):143–9.
64. Webborn N, Cushman D, Blauwet CA, et al. The epidemiology of injuries in football at the London 2012 Paralympic games. PM R 2016;8(6):545–52.
65. Peric M, Zenic N, Sekulic D, et al. Disordered eating, amenorrhea, and substance use and misuse among professional ballet dancers: Preliminary analysis. Med Pregl 2016;67(1):21–7.
66. Robbeson JG, Kruger HS, Wright HH. Disordered eating behavior, body image, and energy status of female student dancers. Int J Sport Nutr Exerc Metab 2015; 25(4):344–52.
67. Padham M, Aujla I. The relationship between passion and the psychological well-being of professional dancers. J Dance Med Sci 2014;18(1):37–44.
68. Brook EM, Tenforde AS, Broad EM, et al. Low energy availability, menstrual dysfunction, and impaired bone health: a survey of elite para athletes. Scand J Med Sci Sport 2019;29(5):678–85.
69. Elson LE. Performing arts medicine. 1st edition. St. Louis: Elsevier; 2018.

Moving?

Make sure your subscription moves with you!

To notify us of your new address, find your **Clinics Account Number** (located on your mailing label above your name), and contact customer service at:

Email: journalscustomerservice-usa@elsevier.com

800-654-2452 (subscribers in the U.S. & Canada)
314-447-8871 (subscribers outside of the U.S. & Canada)

Fax number: 314-447-8029

Elsevier Health Sciences Division
Subscription Customer Service
3251 Riverport Lane
Maryland Heights, MO 63043

*To ensure uninterrupted delivery of your subscription, please notify us at least 4 weeks in advance of move.

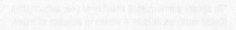

Printed and bound by CPI Group (UK) Ltd, Croydon, CR0 4YY

03/10/2024

01040483-0003

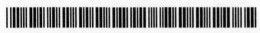